Anomalies of the Developing Dentition

Jane Ann Soxman
Patrice Barsamian Wunsch
Christel M. Haberland

Anomalies of the Developing Dentition

A Clinical Guide to Diagnosis and Management

Springer

Jane Ann Soxman
Private Practice
Allison Park, PA
USA

Christel M. Haberland
Division of Pediatric Dentistry
Johns Hopkins All Children's Hospital
Saint Petersburg, FL
USA

Patrice Barsamian Wunsch
Department of Pediatric Dentistry
Virginia Commonwealth University School of Dentistry
Richmond, VA
USA

ISBN 978-3-030-03163-3 ISBN 978-3-030-03164-0 (eBook)
https://doi.org/10.1007/978-3-030-03164-0

Library of Congress Control Number: 2018962929

This Springer imprint is published by the registered company Springer Nature Switzerland AG
The registered company address is: Gewerbestrasse 11, 6330 Cham, Switzerland

Preface

Once writing began, with photographs and radiographs of the various anomalies being gathered, a heightened awareness resulted in a realization of the frequency of occurrence and combinations of dental anomalies. Thoroughness of the examination is confirmed as clinicians identify an anomaly. Patients and caregivers may have previously noticed the anomaly and appreciate our knowledge of the etiology and its management. During an oral examination, this discussion typically peaks more interest than oral hygiene, caries, or other issues and provides an opportunity for improved interaction.

Developmental anomalies may occur simultaneously and in different combinations. Patterns of association occur with a spectrum of dental anomalies. Because dental anomalies may be associated with many syndromes, awareness of the phenotypic expression of certain anomalies may alert clinicians to the possibility of a genetic trait not yet expressed in a medical history or clinically apparent. The mission of this handbook is to provide a succinct and informative means for healthcare professionals to identify, discuss, and appropriately manage the more common developmental dental anomalies.

Allison Park, PA, USA — Jane Ann Soxman

Contents

1 Tooth Development 1
1.1 Introduction 1
1.2 Physiologic Processes 4
1.2.1 Initiation 4
1.2.2 Proliferation 4
1.2.3 Histodifferentiation 4
1.2.4 Morphodifferentiation 5
1.2.5 Apposition 5
References 6

2 Anomalies of Crown Size 7
2.1 Introduction 7
2.2 Microdontia 7
2.2.1 Description 7
2.2.2 Etiology 9
2.2.3 Treatment/Management 10
2.3 Macrodontia 12
2.3.1 Description 12
2.3.2 Etiology 13
2.3.3 Treatment/Management 13
References 14

3 Anomalies of Crown Shape 15
3.1 Introduction 15
3.2 Pegged Lateral Incisors 15
3.2.1 Description 15
3.2.2 Etiology 16
3.2.3 Treatment/Management 16
3.3 Shovel Incisors 17
3.3.1 Description 17
3.3.2 Etiology 17
3.3.3 Treatment/Management 18

3.4 Accessory Cusps . . . 18
3.4.1 Description . . . 18
3.4.2 Etiology . . . 21
3.4.3 Treatment/Management . . . 21
3.5 Taurodontism . . . 22
3.5.1 Description . . . 22
3.5.2 Etiology . . . 23
3.5.3 Treatment/Management . . . 23
3.6 Mesiodens . . . 24
3.6.1 Description . . . 24
3.6.2 Etiology . . . 26
3.6.3 Treatment/Management . . . 28
References . . . 28

4 Anomalies of Tooth Number . . . 29
4.1 Introduction . . . 29
4.2 Hypodontia/Anodontia . . . 29
4.2.1 Description . . . 29
4.2.2 Etiology . . . 32
4.2.3 Treatment/Management . . . 33
4.3 Hyperdontia/Supernumerary Teeth . . . 40
4.3.1 Description . . . 40
4.3.2 Etiology . . . 42
4.3.3 Treatment/Management . . . 42
References . . . 42

5 Anomalies of Tooth Eruption . . . 45
5.1 Introduction . . . 45
5.2 Natal/Neonatal Teeth . . . 45
5.2.1 Description . . . 45
5.2.2 Etiology . . . 46
5.2.3 Treatment/Management . . . 46
5.3 Ankylosis/Deep Submersion of Primary Molars . . . 47
5.3.1 Description . . . 47
5.3.2 Etiology . . . 49
5.3.3 Treatment/Management . . . 49
5.4 Ectopic Eruption of Maxillary First Permanent Molars . . . 51
5.4.1 Description . . . 51
5.4.2 Etiology . . . 52
5.4.3 Treatment/Management . . . 53
5.5 Ectopic Eruption and Impaction of Maxillary Permanent Canines . . . 61
5.5.1 Description . . . 61
5.5.2 Etiology . . . 62
5.5.3 Treatment/Management . . . 66

5.6 Dental Transposition 70
5.6.1 Description. 70
5.6.2 Etiology 71
5.6.3 Treatment/Management. 71
References. 72

6 Anomalies of Tooth Formation 75
6.1 Introduction 75
6.2 Pre-eruptive Intracoronal Resorption (PEIR) 75
6.2.1 Description. 75
6.2.2 Etiology 76
6.2.3 Treatment/Management. 77
6.3 Ectopic Enamel (Enamel Pearl, Cervical Enamel Extension). 77
6.3.1 Description. 77
6.3.2 Etiology 79
6.3.3 Treatment/Management. 79
6.4 Dens in Dente (Dens Invaginatus). 80
6.4.1 Description. 80
6.4.2 Etiology 83
6.4.3 Treatment/Management. 83
6.5 Gemination. 83
6.5.1 Description. 83
6.5.2 Etiology 84
6.5.3 Management/Treatment. 84
6.6 Fusion. 85
6.6.1 Description. 85
6.6.2 Etiology 87
6.6.3 Management/Treatment. 87
6.7 Concrescence 87
6.7.1 Description. 87
6.7.2 Etiology 89
6.7.3 Treatment 89
6.8 Regional Odontodysplasia 89
6.8.1 Description. 89
6.8.2 Etiology 91
6.8.3 Treatment/Management. 91
6.9 Odontoma. 92
6.9.1 Description. 92
6.9.2 Etiology 93
6.9.3 Treatment/Management. 93
6.10 Molar Root-Incisor Malformation 93
6.10.1 Description. 93
6.10.2 Etiology 94
6.10.3 Treatment/Management. 96

6.11 Dilaceration 96
6.11.1 Description 96
6.11.2 Etiology 97
6.11.3 Treatment/Management 98
6.12 Short Root Anomaly 98
6.12.1 Description 98
6.12.2 Etiology 100
6.12.3 Treatment/Management 100
6.13 Accessory Roots (Supernumerary Roots) 101
6.13.1 Description 101
6.13.2 Etiology 102
6.13.3 Treatment/Management 103
References 103

7 Anomalies of Enamel Formation 109
7.1 Introduction 109
7.2 Hereditary Amelogenesis Imperfecta 110
7.2.1 Description 110
7.2.2 Etiology (Four Types of AI) 110
7.2.3 Treatment/Management 113
7.3 Molar Incisor Hypomineralization (MIH) 114
7.3.1 Description 114
7.3.2 Etiology 114
7.3.3 Treatment/Management 115
7.4 Enamel Hypoplasia/Turner's Tooth 116
7.4.1 Description 116
7.4.2 Etiology 117
7.4.3 Treatment/Management 118
7.5 Opaque Enamel Spots 118
7.5.1 Description 118
7.5.2 Etiology 120
7.5.3 Treatment 120
References 120

8 Anomalies of Dentin Formation 123
8.1 Introduction 123
8.2 Dentinogenesis Imperfecta 125
8.2.1 Description 125
8.3 Classification of Dentinogenesis Imperfecta 126
8.3.1 Description and Etiology of Each Subtype 126
8.3.2 Treatment 129

8.4 Dentinal Dysplasia . . . 130
8.4.1 Description . . . 130
8.4.2 Etiology . . . 131
8.4.3 Treatment . . . 131
8.4.4 Note . . . 132
References . . . 132

9 Rare Dental Anomalies . . . 133
9.1 Introduction . . . 133
9.2 Facial (Labial) Talon Cusp . . . 133
9.3 Lobodontia . . . 134
9.4 Globodontia . . . 135
9.5 Radiculomegaly . . . 136
9.6 Solitary Median Maxillary Central Incisor . . . 136
9.7 Pyramidal Molars . . . 138
References . . . 139

About the Authors

Jane Ann Soxman, BS, RN, DDS graduated from Virginia Commonwealth University School of Dentistry in 1980. Specialty training in Pediatric Dentistry was completed at Children's Hospital of Pittsburgh. She is board certified by the American Board of Pediatric Dentistry and a Fellow in both the American Academy of Pediatric Dentistry and the American College of Dentists. She holds an appointment as voluntary Adjunct Assistant Professor of Pediatric Dentistry in the University of Pittsburgh School of Dental Medicine, Department of Pediatric Dentistry, and is a seminar instructor for general practice residencies at Allegheny General Hospital and the Veterans Affairs Health Care System. Dr. Soxman is Pediatrics Advisor on the advisory board, a column contributor, and manuscript reviewer for *General Dentistry.* She has authored numerous articles in the dental literature and is editor of the *Handbook of Clinical Techniques in Pediatric Dentistry*. She has maintained a private practice in Pediatric Dentistry in Allison Park, Pennsylvania, since 1983. As a national speaker for over 25 years, she is recognized as a leader in continuing education.

Patrice Barsamian Wunsch, BS, DDS, MS is a Professor in the Department of Pediatric Dentistry, School of Dentistry, Virginia Commonwealth University (VCU), where she served as Director of Advanced Education in Pediatric Dentistry from 2011 to 2015. She currently serves as Vice Chair within the Department of Pediatric Dentistry at VCU. Her hospital appointments include VCU Medical Center and Children's Hospital of Richmond at VCU. Dr. Wunsch is board certified by the American Board of Pediatric Dentistry. She received her dental degree from Marquette University, Milwaukee, WI, in 1986. She obtained a Master of Science in Oral Biology and Certificate in Pediatric Dentistry from the University of Maryland, Baltimore, in 2002 and a Fellowship in Pediatric Dentistry from the same university in 2003. Her areas of expertise and interest are early childhood caries, pulp therapy, access to care, and teaching methods to enhance the education of adult learners. Dr. Wunsch has served as an editorial board member for the journal *Pediatric Dentistry*, the official publication of the American Academy of Pediatric Dentistry.

Christel M. Haberland, DDS, MS was born in Guatemala City, Guatemala, where she attended dental school at Universidad Francisco Marroquin. She completed a residency in Oral and Maxillofacial Pathology with an MS degree at Ohio

State University in 1998 and continued on to obtain her US dental degree. She taught Oral Pathology as an Assistant Professor at Temple University from 2000 to 2002. Later, she completed a residency in Pediatric Dentistry at Yale-New Haven Hospital from 2007 to 2009 and subsequently became an assistant clinical instructor. She is board certified in both Oral and Maxillofacial Pathology and Pediatric Dentistry. In 2012, Dr. Haberland started an Oral and Maxillofacial Pathology Biopsy Service in the Department of Pathology, Yale School of Medicine, where she held appointments both in the Department of Pathology and Department of Dentistry at Yale-New Haven Hospital. In 2015, she was appointed the Program Director for the Pediatric Dentistry Residency. She moved to St. Petersburg, Florida, in 2018, to start a Pediatric Dental Program and residency at Johns Hopkins All Children's Hospital. Her interests are in pediatric oral pathology, and she has lectured nationally on this topic.

Tooth Development

1

1.1 Introduction

Anomalies of the developing dentition occur due to absence or interruption of normal tooth development along with genetic and/or environment influences. Size, shape, number, eruption, formation, and the composition of enamel and dentin are reflected in an aberration of development. The genetic control of dental development represents a complex series of events that include both the type, size, and position of the enamel organ and the processes of formation of enamel and dentin [1]. The developmental stages and physiologic processes of odontogenesis provide the knowledge for the time line and origins of the various anomalies.

Dental anomalies may occur independently and often are associated with other anomalies (Figs. 1.1, 1.2, 1.3, and 1.4) and particularly with syndromes (Fig. 1.5) [2]. Each dental anomaly has beginnings during specific stages of tooth development.

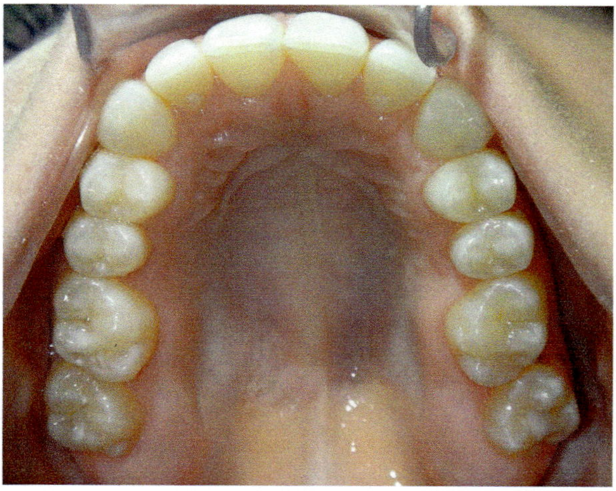

Fig. 1.1 Talon cusps on maxillary right and left permanent lateral incisors

J. A. Soxman et al., *Anomalies of the Developing Dentition*,
https://doi.org/10.1007/978-3-030-03164-0_1

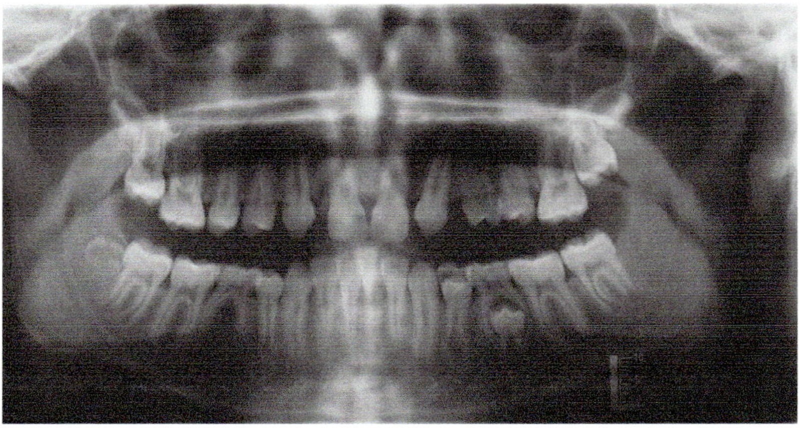

Fig. 1.2 Panoramic radiograph revealing multiple anomalies with agenesis of maxillary right and left permanent lateral incisors, mandibular right second premolar, and left third molar

Fig. 1.3 Clinical photograph showing shovel maxillary permanent central incisors and large talon cusp maxillary permanent left lateral incisor

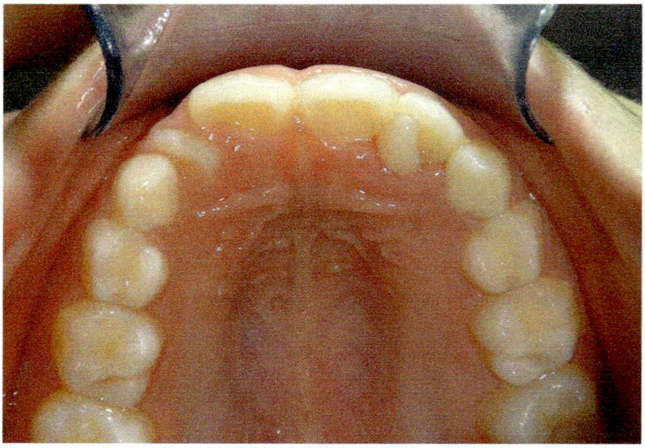

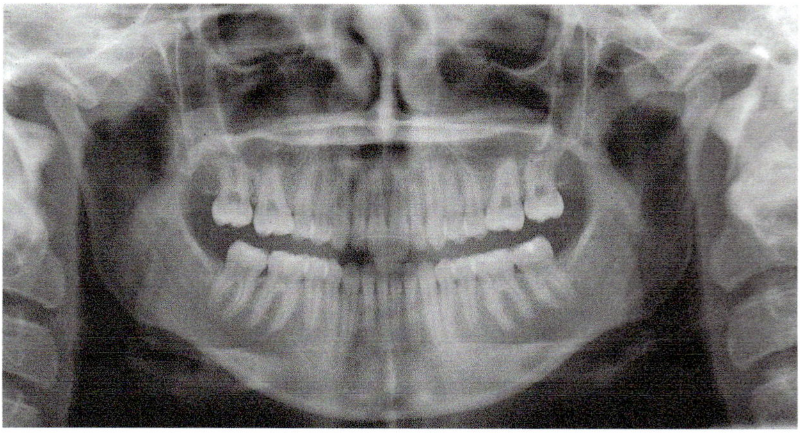

Fig. 1.4 Panoramic radiograph revealing agenesis of all four third molars, microdontia maxillary right and left permanent lateral incisors, and pyramidal maxillary right and left permanent first molars

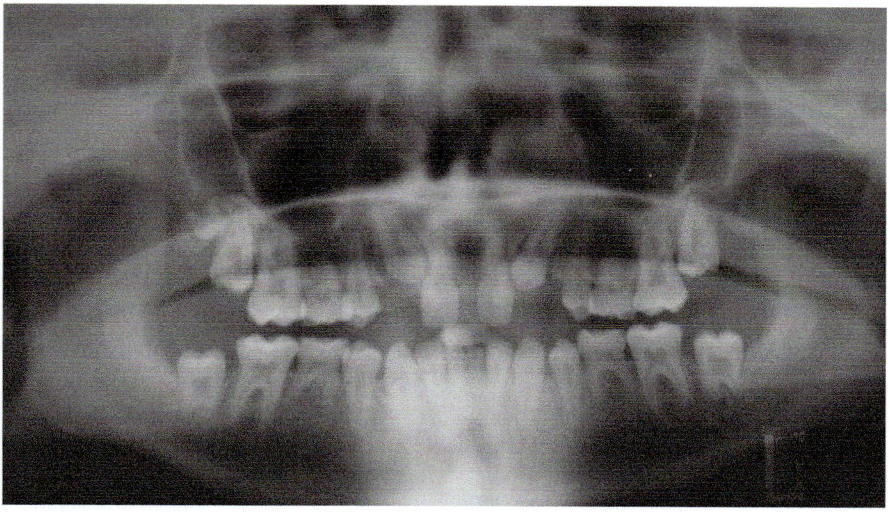

Fig. 1.5 Panoramic radiograph revealing multiple anomalies in Down syndrome with microdontia of maxillary right third molar, agenesis of multiple permanent teeth, ectopic eruption of maxillary right and left permanent canines, and developing taurodontism mandibular right and left permanent second molars

Table 1.1 Stages in tooth growth showing overlap of the various physiologic processes and morphologic stages of tooth development with the exception of the initiation stage
Reprinted by permission [3]

Morphologic stages	Physiologic processes
Dental lamina ←——→	Initiation
Bud stage	
Cap stage	—— Proliferation
Bell stage (early)	—— Histodifferentiation
Bell stage (advanced)	—— Morphodifferentiation
Formation of enamel and dentin matrix	—— Apposition

Physiologic processes include Initiation, Proliferation, Histodifferentiation, Morphodifferentiation, and Apposition [3]. Central features of dental development are the formation of the epithelial placode, the budding of the epithelium, the condensation of mesenchyme around the bud, and the folding and growth of the epithelium generating the shape of the tooth crown [4]. The developmental stages of Bud, Cap, Bell, and Advanced Bell Stage are termed as the Morphologic stages of tooth growth. With the exception of initiation, physiologic processes of development overlap during the morphologic stages of tooth growth as shown in Table 1.1. Teeth form from the surface ectoderm of the first branchial arch and the frontonasal prominence as well as from the underlying mesenchyme that is derived from the neural crest. Therefore, the first branchial arch epithelium is necessary for tooth development, and multiple genes are involved in tooth formation [1, 4]. The genes that regulate tooth development have been researched extensively and to date over 300 genes have been associated with the patterning and morphogenesis as well as with cell differentiation in teeth [4].

1.2 Physiologic Processes

1.2.1 Initiation

Initiation of tooth development begins in the fifth week of embryonic development [3]. The dental lamina exists in a part of the oral epithelium with the potential for tooth formation. Specific cells in the dental lamina contain the growth potential to form specific teeth, and will initiate formation at different times, when directed by the factors that initiate tooth development. Ectodermal cells in the dental lamina rapidly multiply at certain points and form the beginning of the enamel organs, as they grow into the underlying mesenchyme. The enamel organs do not develop simultaneously as they give rise to the primary dentition and later to the permanent dentition. The first enamel organ appears in the mandibular incisor area. The permanent molars arise from a distal extension of the dental lamina, as the jaws grow distally. The succedaneous teeth form between 20 weeks in utero (permanent central incisor) and 10 months postpartum (second premolar). The first permanent molar begins formation at 20 weeks in utero and the third molar at 5 years of age [3, 5]. Disruption during initiation results in congenitally missing teeth. The teeth most often missing due to lack of initiation are maxillary lateral incisors, third molars, and mandibular second premolars. Anodontia results from generalized lack of initiation. Abnormal initiation may also result in development of one or many supernumerary teeth [3] (as discussed in Chap. 4).

1.2.2 Proliferation

Proliferation follows the momentary event of initiation and is divided into stages for descriptive purposes. These include the bud, cap bell (early and advanced), and formation of the enamel and dentin matrix. The development of the tooth germs is initiated during the bud stage. At ten different locations, each corresponding to the future position of the primary dentition, round or ovoid swellings arise from the basement membrane to become the tooth buds. Certain epithelial cells in the tooth bud will ultimately form tooth enamel. Consequently, the enamel organ is formed during the bud stage. Around the ninth week of embryonic development, proliferation of cells in different areas of the tooth bud results in the cap stage, formed by a shallow invagination on the lower surface of each bud. Although each tooth goes through similar stages of development, the shape and size varies according to the location in the dental arch. The size and proportions of the growing tooth germ are the result of proliferative growth [3, 5].

1.2.3 Histodifferentiation

Histodifferentiation follows proliferation, occurring in the same stages as proliferation. Now, the formative cells, developed during proliferation, undergo morphologic and functional modifications and acquire their appositional growth potential for formation of the enamel and dentin matrix. The potency of the cells becomes restricted and they can no longer multiply. The highest development of histodifferentiation occurs in the advanced bell stage when the future dentinoenamel junction is formed by the boundary between inner enamel epithelium and odontoblasts. Dentin formation precedes and is essential to the formation of enamel. After formation of dentin, the cells of the inner enamel epithelium differentiate into ameloblasts [3].

1.2.4 Morphodifferentiation

Morphodifferentiation, occurring during the same morphologic stages as proliferation and histodifferentiation, establishes the form and size of the future tooth with differential growth. Without proliferation, morphodifferentiation cannot occur. Disturbances during morphodifferentiation may present with clinical features such as macrodontia, microdontia, malformed teeth, taurodontism, dens invaginatus, supernumerary cusps or roots, and gemination, along with absent cusps or roots (as discussed in Chaps. 2, 3, 4, 6, and 9). Since functions of odontoblasts and ameloblasts are not affected, dentin and enamel are normal. Endocrine disturbances in utero or during the first year of life effect the size and shape of the crown. Root morphology is affected with disturbance during later periods [3, 5, 6, 7]. During the advanced bell stage, mineralization and root development begin. At this time, enamel and dentin formation have reached the future cementoenamel junction. After crown formation is complete, the cervical portion of the enamel organ contributes to the formation of Hertwig's epithelial root sheath (HERS). HERS determines the shape, length, size, and number of roots via proliferation of the epithelial cells of the inner and outer enamel epithelium. HERS cells influence the differentiation of the radicular dental papilla cells into odontoblasts, which lay down the first layer of dentin in the roots. This dentin is continuous with coronal dentin. Once the first layer of dentin is formed, HERS begins to lose its structural continuity. Enamel pearls, usually located in the furcation of a permanent molar's roots, are the result of HERS cells remaining on the dentin surface that differentiated into ameloblasts, forming enamel. Dilaceration results from distortion of HERS due to injury or pressure (as discussed in Chap. 6). A failure of HERS to invaginate at the proper level has been implicated in taurodontism [3, 5] (as discussed in Chap. 3). With the loss of the epithelium on the dentin surface, connective tissue cells of the dental sac come in contact with the outer layer of dentin, differentiate into cementoblasts, and deposit a layer of cementum. HERS disintegrates. Division of the root trunk into two or three roots occurs with differential growth of the epithelial diaphragm.

1.2.5 Apposition

Apposition occurs with the deposition of enamel, dentin, and cementum, deposited in a layer-like matrix that is incapable of further growth. This stage is the completion of the plan outlined by histodifferentiation and morphodifferentiation. Clinical features of disturbances during apposition include anomalies of enamel and dentin formation (as discussed in Chaps. 7 and 8). If mineralization of a normal organic matrix is defective, the result is hypocalcification or hypomineralization of enamel or dentin. Genetic and environmental influences may affect normal formation of the enamel matrix, resulting in enamel hypoplasia [3]. Examples of disruption during histodifferentiation, apposition, and mineralization are found with amelogenesis imperfecta, dentinogenesis imperfecta, and dentinal dysplasia [6, 7].

References

1. Bailleul-Forestier I, Molla M, Verloes A, Berdal A (2008) The genetic basis of inherited anomalies of the teeth. Part 1: clinical and molecular aspects of non-syndromic dental disorders. Eur J Med Genet 51(4):273–291
2. Bailleul-Forestier I, Berdal A, Vinckier F, de Ravel T, Fryns JP, Verloes A (2008) The genetic basis of inherited anomalies of the teeth. Part 2: syndromes with significant dental involvement. Eur J Med Genet 51(5):383–408
3. Kumar GS (2011) In: Bhaskar SN (ed) Orban's oral histology and embryology, 13th edn. Elsevier, New Delhi, p 37
4. Thesleff I (2006) The genetic basis of tooth development and dental defects. Am J Med Genet A 140(23):2530–2535
5. Nanci A (2013) Ten Cate's oral histology, 8th edn. Elsevier, St. Louis
6. American Academy of Pediatric Dentistry (2017) Dental management of heritable dental developmental anomalies. Pediatr Dent 39(6):348–353
7. Thesleff I (2014) Current understanding of the process of tooth formation: transfer from the laboratory to the clinic. Aust Dent J 59(Suppl 1):48–54

Anomalies of Crown Size

2

2.1 Introduction

Anomalies of crown size are commonly encountered in the dentition. Disruption during the morphogenic stage of tooth formation can result in one, multiple, or all teeth presenting with this anomaly. Various factors including genetics, environmental influences, chemotherapy, irradiation, and syndromes may be responsible for anomalies of crown size. Treatment may involve multiple disciplines.

2.2 Microdontia

2.2.1 Description

The tooth crown is smaller in size than normal or relative to other teeth. Isolated microdontia is the typical presentation, involving one or two teeth. Teeth most often affected are lateral incisors and third molars (Figs. 2.1 and 2.2) [1, 2]. The prevalence of microdontia of the maxillary permanent lateral incisors is from 0.8 to 8.4% [2]. Microdontia of lateral incisors may also be termed as pegged or peg-shaped. The mesiodistal width is smaller, narrowing to the incisal edge and often ending in a point (Fig. 2.3). Microdontia of a permanent lateral incisor is often associated with a congenitally missing permanent lateral incisor in the same arch (Fig. 2.4). Microdontia of second premolars does occur, but less frequently (Fig. 2.5) [3]. Diffuse or true generalized microdontia presents with every tooth smaller than normal. Relative microdontia describes teeth of normal size that are widely spaced in the maxilla and mandible due to macrognathia [2]. Heredity plays a role in this presentation with the offspring inheriting large jaws from one parent and teeth of normal size from the other parent. Although esthetics is the most common complaint, food impaction and malocclusion are also cited. Palatal impaction of the maxillary permanent canine has also been associated with microdontia [4]. Microdontia is often associated with hypodontia, with females exhibiting a higher incidence of microdontia and hypodontia [2].

J. A. Soxman et al., *Anomalies of the Developing Dentition*,
https://doi.org/10.1007/978-3-030-03164-0_2

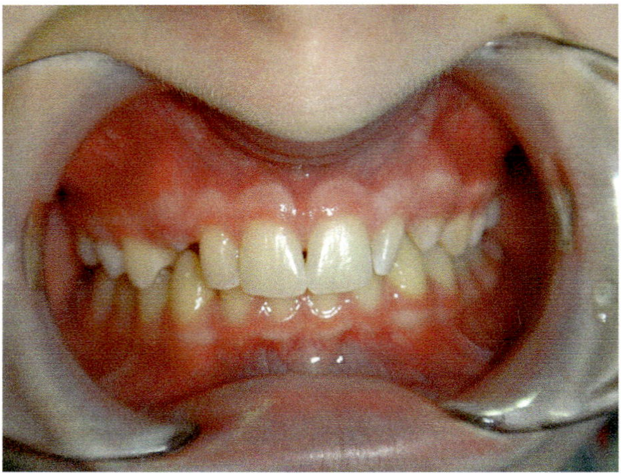

Fig. 2.1 Clinical photograph showing microdontia of maxillary right and left permanent lateral incisors

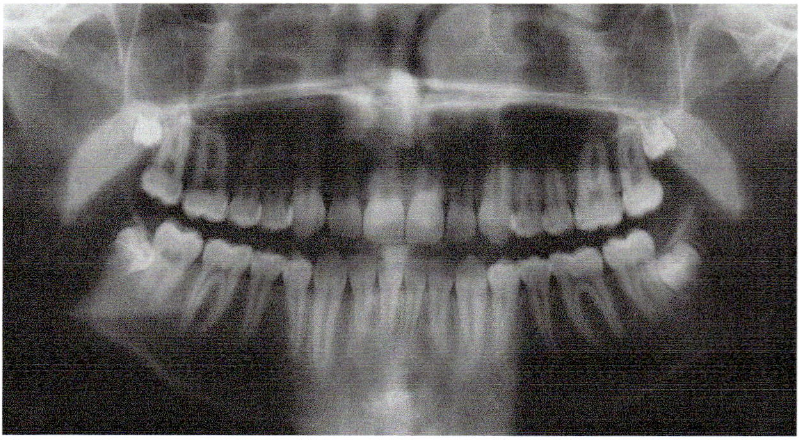

Fig. 2.2 Panoramic radiograph revealing microdontia of maxillary right third molar

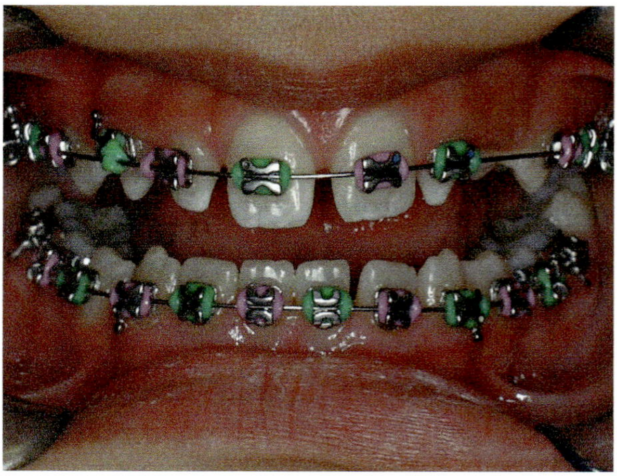

Fig. 2.3 Clinical photograph showing pegged maxillary left permanent lateral incisor

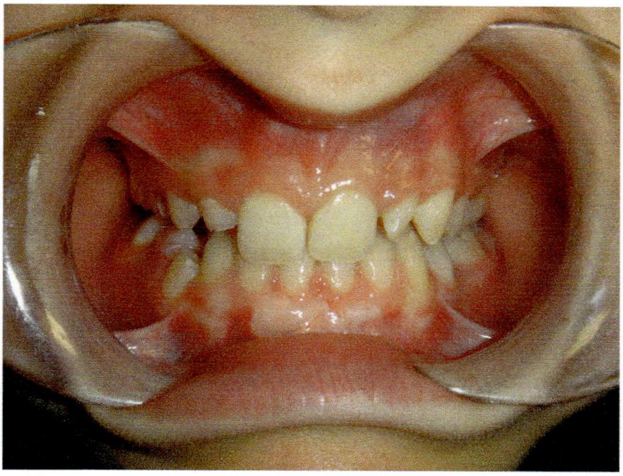

Fig. 2.4 Clinical photograph showing missing maxillary right permanent lateral incisor and microdontia of maxillary left permanent lateral incisor

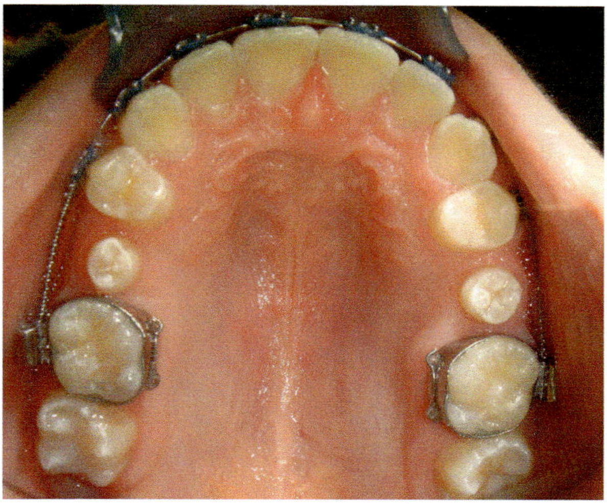

Fig. 2.5 Clinical photograph showing microdontia of maxillary right and left second premolars

2.2.2 Etiology

A disruption during the physiologic process of morphodifferentiation during the bell stage of tooth development, when the blueprint for the individual size and shape of teeth is created, results in anomalies of crown size [1, 5]. Disturbances during morphodifferentiation typically do not impair function of the ameloblasts or odontoblasts; so enamel and dentin are normal [4].

Heredity is reported as autosomal dominant with incomplete penetrance in isolated microdontia [2]. Isolated or spontaneous cases have been reported where no etiology has been identified [4]. True generalized microdontia rarely occurs, but has been reported in children after chemotherapy or radiation therapy during tooth development and with Fanconi's anemia. Other associated syndromes include Gorlin–Chaudhry–Moss syndrome, Williams's syndrome, Ullrich–Turner syndrome, Rothmund–Thomson syndrome, Hallermann–Streiff, and orofaciodigital syndrome [4]. Down syndrome and pituitary dwarfism are also associated with diffuse or true generalized microdontia [2]. Microdontia may be associated with other disorders and anomalies such as dens invaginatus, fourth molars, oligodontia, hereditary hypohidrotic ectodermal dysplasia, chondroectodermal dysplasia (Ellis–van Creveld), hemifacial microsomia, and Crouzon's disease [2].

Chemotherapy and cranial or total body radiation can interfere with dental development, resulting in multiple dental anomalies. High-dose chemotherapy under 4 years of age is a risk factor for microdontia and tooth agenesis [6]. Javed et al. found 100% of children under 5 years of age, treated with chemotherapy and cranial irradiation, exhibited dental anomalies such as microdontia, arrested root development, enamel dysplasia, and tooth agenesis [7].

2.2.3 Treatment/Management

Treatment is typically targeted to correct the esthetic issues presenting with microdontia of a permanent lateral incisor. If the mesiodistal width of the lateral incisor is esthetically acceptable, no intervention or minor orthodontic space closure may be necessary (Figs. 2.6 and 2.7). If the size and shape of the lateral and the excessive spacing between the teeth are of concern, a number of treatment options can be offered. These options typically require multidisciplinary involvement that may include restorative, prosthetic, orthodontic, or surgical intervention.

Treatment options include:

- Restorative treatment options may include direct composite resin crowns, ceramic or composite veneers, all-ceramic crowns, and porcelain-fused-to metal crowns. Vertical positioning of the pegged lateral may determine the position of

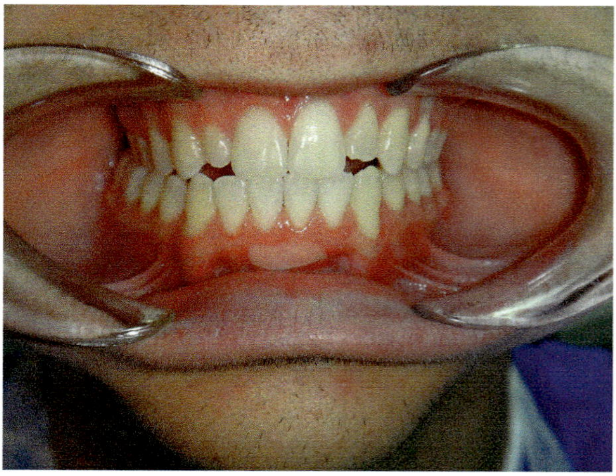

Fig. 2.6 Clinical photograph showing esthetically acceptable microdontia of maxillary right permanent lateral incisor

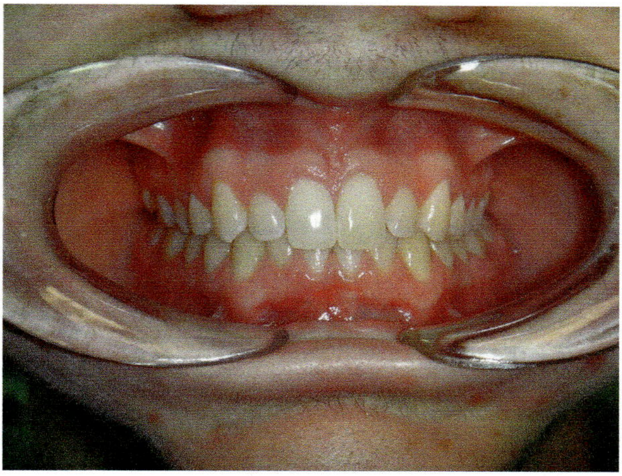

Fig. 2.7 Clinical photograph showing esthetically acceptable mild microdontia of maxillary right and left permanent lateral incisors

the gingival margin and the material selected for restoration [4]. Since growth has not been completed and gingival margins will change, a composite resin crown is the restoration of choice for the pediatric patient. Typically, no preparation of the tooth is required, avoiding any risk of pulpal exposure. As marginal gingival levels move apically, composite can be added. Veneers offer good esthetics and are more conservative with less tooth preparation than porcelain crowns. Veneers may be composite or ceramic. Tooth preparation should be minimal to maintain adequate enamel for optimal retention. If a porcelain veneer is the restoration of choice, the structural integrity of the pegged lateral and adequate thickness of the veneer incisally may be obtained by intruding the tooth apically about 2 mm [4].

- Orthodontic treatment may align the pegged lateral and create the necessary space for an ideal restoration. If the tooth is thick labially, a slightly palatal position of the pegged lateral may be advisable in order to permit adequate thickness of the restoration and avoid labial preparation or a bulky-appearing final restoration [4]. Collaboration between the referring dentist and the orthodontist will determine the space and position necessary for restoration. Closing the space may result in less than acceptable esthetics and adversely alter the posterior occlusion. These limitations should be discussed with the patient. Near the end of orthodontic treatment, the dentist performing the restorative treatment should evaluate the capability of the space and tooth position to accommodate the planned restoration.
- With a poor long-term prognosis, extraction of the pegged lateral incisor may be the optimal treatment choice. Circumstances that may require extraction include severely rotated teeth, teeth with short, thin roots, and crowns that are too short or malformed to restore. Additionally, teeth with anomalies such as amelogenesis imperfecta or dens in dente may require extraction [4]. Canine substitution or orthodontics to open or close space for an implant or a Maryland bridge offers treatment options post-extraction (as discussed in Chap. 4).

2.3 Macrodontia

2.3.1 Description

The tooth crown is larger than typical size for that particular tooth. Alternative terms include megalodontia, megadontia, and gigantism [1, 2]. True macrodontia should not be confused with fused or geminated teeth (Figs. 2.8 and 2.9) (as discussed in Chap. 6). Incidence in the permanent dentition is about 1.1% and is more common in males [1]. Isolated or localized macrodontia occurs most often in incisors (Figs. 2.10 and 2.11) and canines, but has been reported in second premolars and third molars. Diffuse or generalized macrodontia is rare and involves only a few teeth [2, 8].

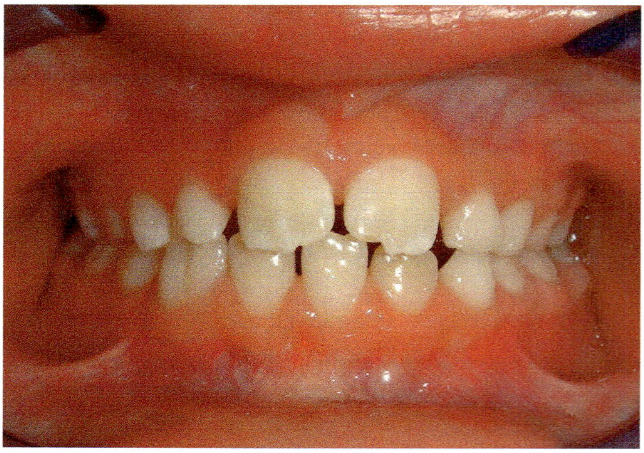

Fig. 2.8 Clinical photograph showing fusion of mandibular right primary lateral incisor and canine

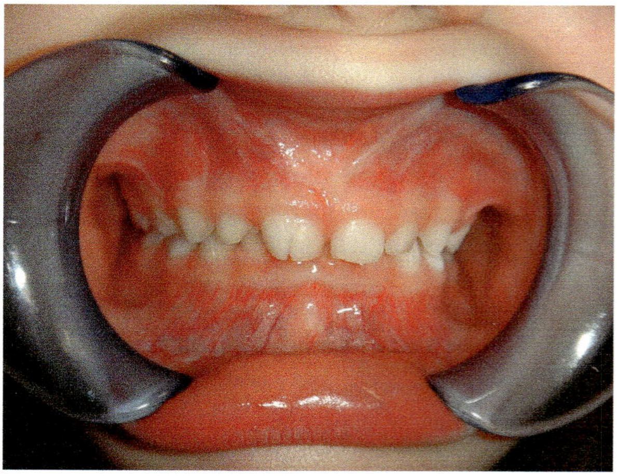

Fig. 2.9 Clinical photograph showing germination of maxillary right primary central incisor

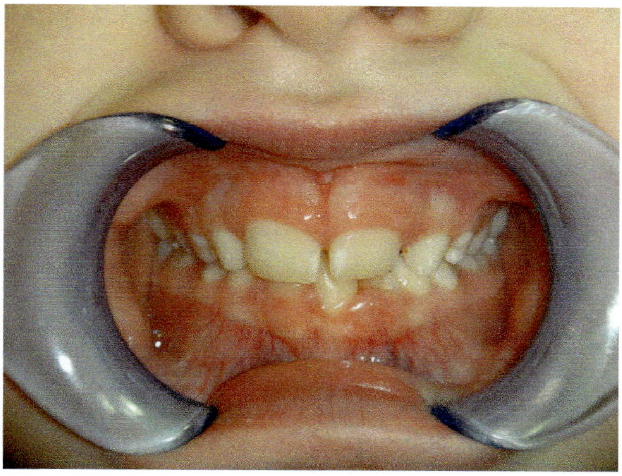

Fig. 2.10 Clinical photograph showing macrodontia of maxillary right and left permanent central incisors

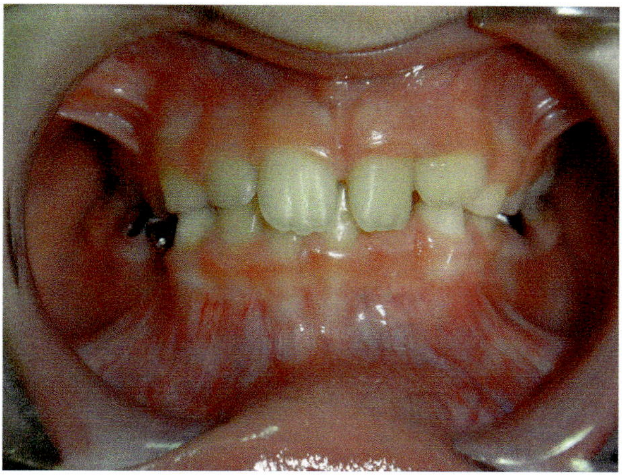

Fig. 2.11 Clinical photograph showing macrodontia of maxillary left permanent lateral incisor

2.3.2 Etiology

Because no genetic component for tooth-size asymmetry has been documented, macrodontia is considered to be the consequence of a phenotypic environmental disturbance during tooth development [8]. Macrodontia has been associated with pituitary gigantism, otodental syndrome, XYY males, hyperinsulinism, pineal hyperplasia, and facial hemihyperplasia [2].

2.3.3 Treatment/Management

- No treatment is necessary unless for esthetic purposes.
- Enameloplasty with interproximal stripping, but minimal change typically occurs and may risk pulp exposure and tooth vitality.

- Extraction of maxillary central incisors with macrodontia and excessive overjet. Orthodontic movement of the lateral incisors into the space for space closure [8].
- Orthodontic intervention for crowding, malocclusion.
- Extraction and replacement with Maryland bridge or implant.
- All factors relating to the stomatognathic system with treatment plan, including malocclusion, and results of treatment must be considered [8].

References

1. Cameron AC, Widmer RP (eds) (2008) Dental anomalies. In: Handbook of pediatric dentistry, 3rd edn. Mosby, London, pp 236–238
2. Laverty DP, Thomas MBM (2016) The restorative management of microdontia. Br Dent J 221:160–166
3. Neville BW, Damm DD, Allen CM, Chi AC (2016) Abnormalities of teeth. In: Oral and maxillofacial pathology, 4th edn. Elsevier, St. Louis, p 76
4. Kumar GS (2011) In: Bhaskar SN (ed) Orban's oral histology and embryology. Elsevier, New Delhi, p 46
5. Ten Cate AR, Nanci A, (2013) Ten Cate's oral histology. Elsevier, St. Louis p 82
6. Nishimura S, Inada H, Sawa Y et al (2013) Risk factors to cause tooth formation anomalies in chemotherapy of paediatric cancers. Eur J Cancer Care 22(3):353–360
7. Javed F, Utreja A, Correa FOB et al (2012) Oral health status in children with acute lymphoblastic leukemia. Crit Rev Oncol Hematol 83:303–309
8. Hellekant M, Twetman S, Carlsson L (2001) Treatment of a class II division I malocclusion with macrodontia of the maxillary incisors. Am J Orthod Dentofac Orthop 119(6):654–659

Anomalies of Crown Shape

3

3.1 Introduction

A disruption during the morphodifferentiation stage of tooth development results in anomalies of crown shape. Multiple factors such as chromosomal abnormalities, mutations, environmental forces, and traumatic injury may be responsible for anomalies of crown shape.

3.2 Pegged Lateral Incisors

3.2.1 Description

As discussed in Chap. 2, pegged lateral is another term to describe a crown that is smaller than the norm and cone-shaped with a root that is normal in length (Fig. 3.1).

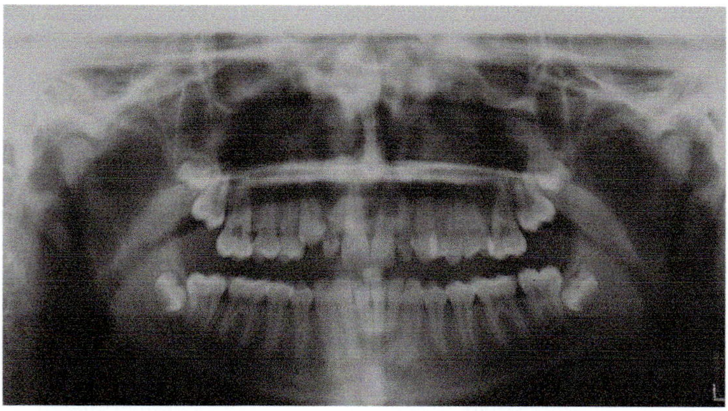

Fig. 3.1 Panoramic radiograph revealing pegged maxillary right and left permanent lateral incisors (also noted pyramidal first permanent molars)

J. A. Soxman et al., *Anomalies of the Developing Dentition*,
https://doi.org/10.1007/978-3-030-03164-0_3

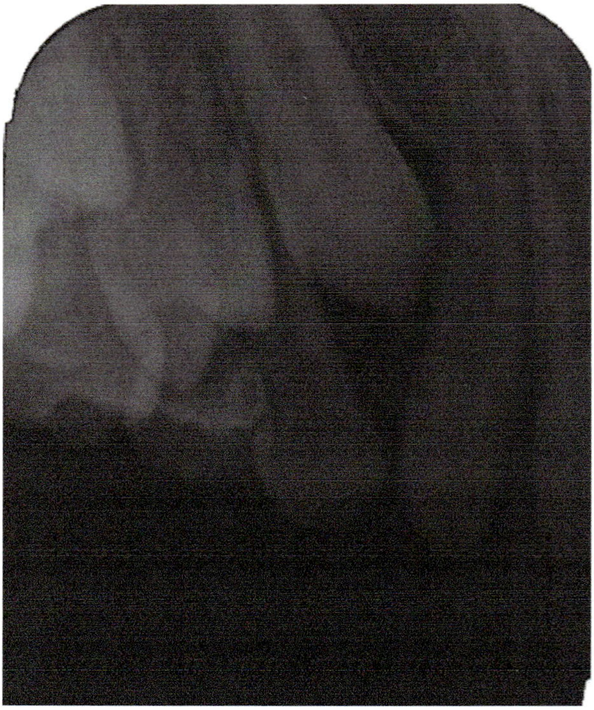

Fig. 3.2 Periapical radiograph revealing pegged maxillary permanent lateral incisor associated with ectopic maxillary permanent canine

The remaining dentition may be smaller mesiodistally. Pegged lateral incisors are associated with palatally displaced and ectopic maxillary permanent canines (Fig. 3.2) [1]. A maxillary midline diastema is often present due to distal movement of the central incisor. Other anomalies associated with pegged lateral incisors are taurodontism, rotated premolars, and canine transposition [2].

3.2.2 Etiology

Environmental and genetic factors impact the size of the developing dentition; however, heredity is the major factor [3]. This anomaly occurs via an autosomal dominant mode of transmission with incomplete penetrance and variation in expression of the trait [2].

3.2.3 Treatment/Management

Treatment, as discussed in Chap. 2, may be performed. A staged approach, usually beginning with orthodontic positioning, is the typical course. Esthetic restoration with a composite resin crown can be performed prior to the final retention phase of orthodontic treatment. In some cases, composite resin crowns may be all that is required to attain a more esthetic appearance in the young patient.

3.3 Shovel Incisors

3.3.1 Description

The term shovel-shaped incisor designates a morphologic form commonly found in the maxillary incisors of some human races. These incisors are characterized by accentuated marginal ridges, surrounding a deep lingual fossa [4]. The condition was first described by Murhlreiter' in 1870 and later Hardlicka classified this anomaly on the basis of the degree of shoveling into three types. The first type is the shovel and shows a thick enamel rim surrounding a well-developed lingual fossa, creating a shovel-like morphology (Fig. 3.3); the second type is the semishovel and shows that the enamel rim is still distinct and encloses a shallower lingual fossa, and the third type is the trace shovel which shows distinct traces of enamel rim but the lingual fossa is shallower than the semishovel type [4]. Central and lateral incisors are most often involved. The anomaly occurs predominately in Asians and nearly 100 per cent in Native Americans and the Inui, and is rare or absent in European and African populations [3, 5]. Rarely, shoveling can occur on the lingual and the labial surfaces at the same time and this has been described as "double shovels" [6].

3.3.2 Etiology

Shoveling is determined primarily by genetic factors. Genes for population-specific phenotypes have been identified. In humans, a dysfunctional mutation in the ectodysplasin A receptor gene (EDAR) in combination with the ectodysplasin A gene (EDA) causes hypohidrotic ectodermal dysplasia. This genetic disorder presents as abnormal morphogenesis of teeth, hair, and sweat glands. Hence, a variation in EDAR is a genetic determinant of shovel-shaped incisors [5].

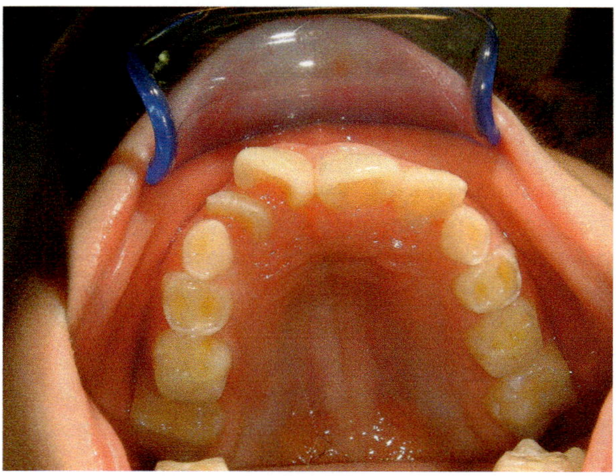

Fig. 3.3 Clinical photograph showing maxillary right and left permanent central and lateral shovel incisors

3.3.3 Treatment/Management

Reshaping of the clinical crown or restorative intervention may be necessary to achieve ideal overjet or overbite with orthodontic treatment. Examination for enamel defects or deep fissures should be performed and a composite restoration or sealant placed to prevent caries ingression to a large, young pulp [3].

3.4 Accessory Cusps

The three most commonly encountered presentations include talon cusp, cusp of Carabelli, and dens evaginatus. Teeth often are slightly larger in dentitions with accessory cusps [3]. These cusps are characterized by an enamel-covered conical tubercle containing dentin and possibly pulpal tissue. With attrition or cuspal fracture, pulpal necrosis may occur due to pulpal extensions. Extra cusps may present other problems such as caries in the pits or developmental fissure between the cusp and the tooth, and sensitivity. Accessory cusps occur in both the primary and the permanent dentitions. In the anterior teeth, the tubercle typically forms on the lingual surface and is referred to as a talon cusp. In the posterior teeth, the tubercle may be found on the central groove of the occlusal surface or the inclined plane of a buccal cusp [7].

3.4.1 Description

3.4.1.1 Talon Cusp

A talon cusp is a cusp-like protuberance from the cingulum on the lingual surface of maxillary incisors, which may be unilateral or bilateral. Most often, the shape of the cusp resembles an eagle's talon. The cusp may extend from the cementoenamel junction to the incisal edge. Three types of talon cusps have been described. In Type 1, the talon is well-delineated, extending at least half the distance from the cementoenamel junction to the incisal edge of a primary or permanent incisor (Fig. 3.4). Type 2 is a semitalon 1 mm or more in size, extending less than half the distance from the cementoenamel junction to the incisal edge. Type 3 is a trace talon that is any of the variant forms of bifid, conical, or tubercle-like and originates from the cervical third of the root. The cusp may blend into the palatal or protrude from the crown [8]. Talon cusp occurs predominately in the permanent dentition with 55% on lateral incisors, 33% on central incisors, and 6% and 4%, respectively, on mandibular incisors and maxillary canines. Various extensions of pulp tissue may extend into the cusp [3, 8]. Alternative terms are T cingulum and Y-shaped cingulum [9]. Talon cusp occurs during early odontogenesis [8]. Genetic influences may be included in the etiology. Occurrence is more frequent in Asians, people of Arab descent, and Artic people also known as the Inuit and Native Americans. Talon cusps occur in various syndromes such as Ellis–van Creveld, incontinentia pigmenti achromians, Mohr, Sturge–Weber angiomatosis, Berardinelli–Seip, and Rubinstein–Taybi, which is most strongly associated with the presence of talon cusps. Parental consanguinity is also associated with talon cusp [8].

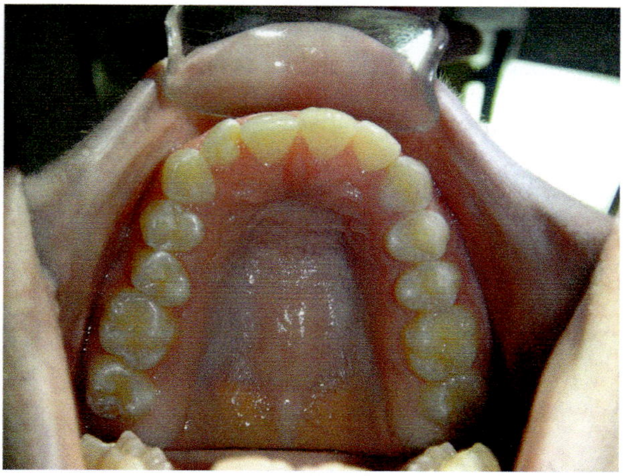

Fig. 3.4 Clinical photograph showing talon cusp maxillary right permanent lateral incisor

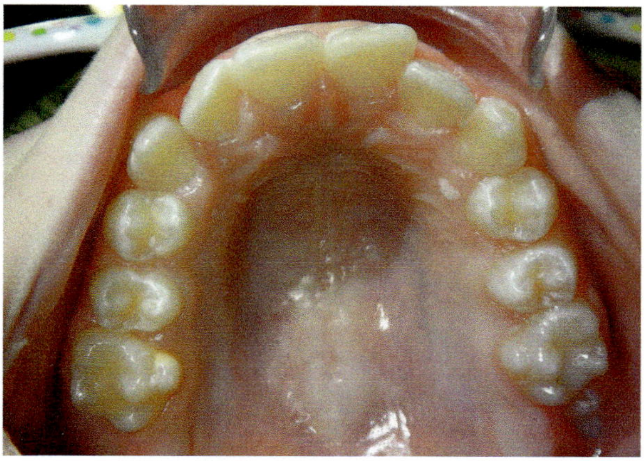

Fig. 3.5 Clinical photograph showing maxillary right permanent first molar with excessively large cusp of Carabelli

3.4.1.2 Cusp of Carabelli

The cusp of Carabelli is located on the mesiolingual surface of maxillary permanent first molar. The size of the cusp varies from a small pit to an excessively large cusp (Fig. 3.5) and gradually decreases in size from the permanent first molar to the third molar. The prevalence is about 90% in Caucasians and rare in the Asian population. A comparable cusp on the mesiobuccal surface of a mandibular permanent first molar is termed a protostylid (Fig. 3.6) [3].

3.4.1.3 Dens Evaginatus

Dens evaginatus presents clinically as a tubercle or elevation of enamel, typically protruding from the occlusal surface bilaterally of a mandibular premolar (Fig. 3.7). This anomaly may also occur on a maxillary premolar and is often associated with shovel-shaped incisors (Fig. 3.8). Pulp tissue may be present within the tubercle in about 43% of teeth. A radiograph should be obtained to determine if pulp extends into tubercle. This anomaly occurs more often bilaterally, in females, Native Americans,

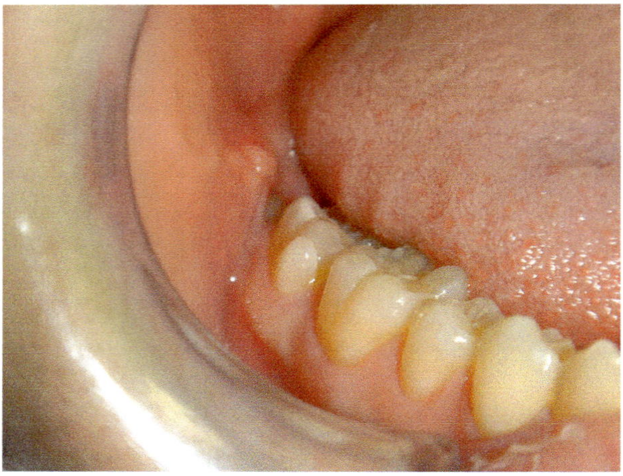

Fig. 3.6 Clinical photograph showing protostylid mesiobuccal surface of mandibular permanent second molar

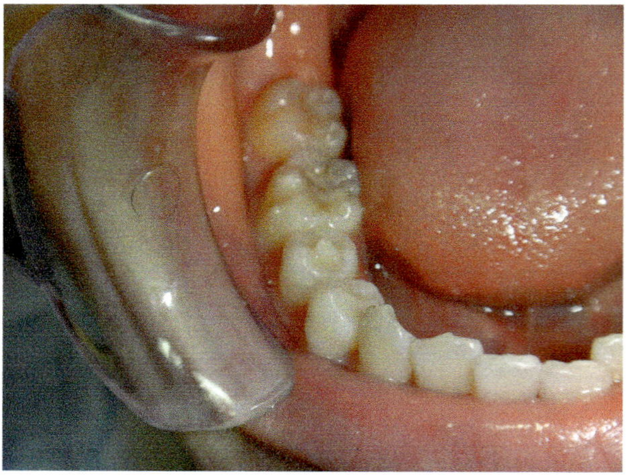

Fig. 3.7 Clinical photograph showing dens evaginatus protruding from occlusal surface of mandibular second premolar

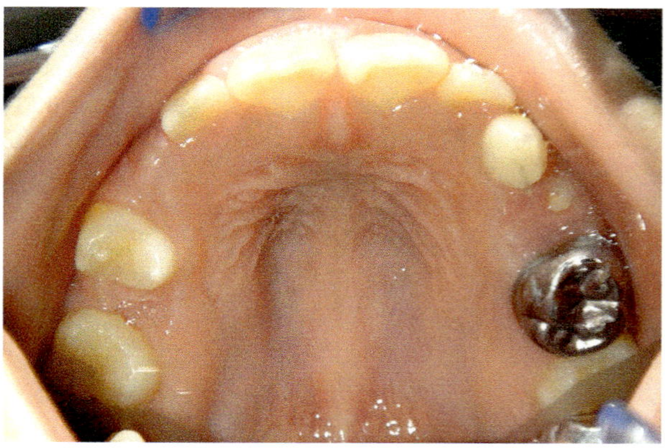

Fig. 3.8 Clinical photograph showing dens evaginatus protruding from occlusal cusp of maxillary premolar associated with maxillary right and left permanent central shovel incisors

the Inuit, and predominately in Asian populations. Dens evaginatus is also termed as central tubercle, accessory tubercle, tuberculated premolar, occlusal enamel pearl, axial core type odontome, composite dilated odontome, cone-shaped supernumerary cusp, evaginated odontome, interstitial cusp, and Leong premolar [3, 9].

3.4.2 Etiology

A disruption during the Bell stage of tooth formation results in an accessory cusp. Abnormal proliferation of a part of the inner enamel epithelium and adjacent ecto-mesenchymal cells of the dental papilla occurs and folds into the stellate reticulum of the enamel organ. The result is a tubercle or supplemental enamel elevation in some area of the crown's surface. Both genetic and environmental influences have been reported, along with parental consanguinity in the case of talon cusps [7, 8].

3.4.3 Treatment/Management

No intervention is usually necessary, but a very prominent talon cusp bulge may cause various clinical problems. An excessively large talon cusp could be mistaken as a supernumerary. A strand of floss can confirm unity of the talon with the incisor (Fig. 3.9). Poor esthetics, attrition of the opposing incisor, displacement of the affected incisor, or cuspal fracture, causing a pulp exposure requiring endodontic intervention can occur. If the talon cusp is in traumatic occlusion, irritating the tongue or would impede attainment of ideal overjet/overbite during orthodontic treatment, cusp reduction is required. Reduction should be performed cautiously, since pulp tissue may be located within the cusp. Gradual enameloplasty may be performed to permit deposition of tertiary dentin and recession of pulp tissue. In some cases, endodontic therapy may be performed before reducing the cusp(s).

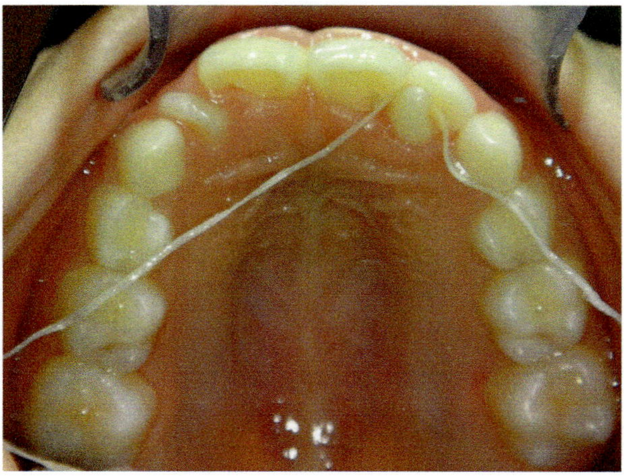

Fig. 3.9 Clinical photograph showing large talon cusp with floss threaded to rule out supernumerary

Application of fluoride varnish will reduce sensitivity during enameloplasty. Exposed dentin can be restored with composite after removal of the cusp [3]. A sealant may be placed to protect developmental grooves from carious involvement [9].

A large cusp of Carabelli may create difficulty in fitting bands for space maintainers or orthodontic treatment. If accompanied by deep grooves, placement of a sealant is advised to protect against caries [3].

Traumatic occlusion with dens evaginatus may cause pulpal necrosis. Enameloplasty may be performed to reduce the cusp, but the risk of pulpal involvement is a concern. Alternatively, the opposing tooth can be reduced to lighten occlusal contact and wait for complete root development should endodontic treatment become necessary [3].

3.5 Taurodontism

3.5.1 Description

The crown of a molar enlarges, resulting in short roots with a bifurcation close to the apex and an elongated, apically displaced floor of the pulp chamber. These teeth are rectangular in shape with less cervical constriction, mimicking the molar morphology of cud-chewing animals. Taurodontism may occur unilaterally or bilaterally and is less prevalent in primary molars. The extent of involvement, determined by the location of the bi- or trifurcation above the root apices, is classified by mild or hypotaurodontism, moderate or mesotaurodontism (Fig. 3.10), and severe or hypertaurodontism (Fig. 3.11). Diagnosis is made radiographically. This anomaly occurs more frequently with cleft lip

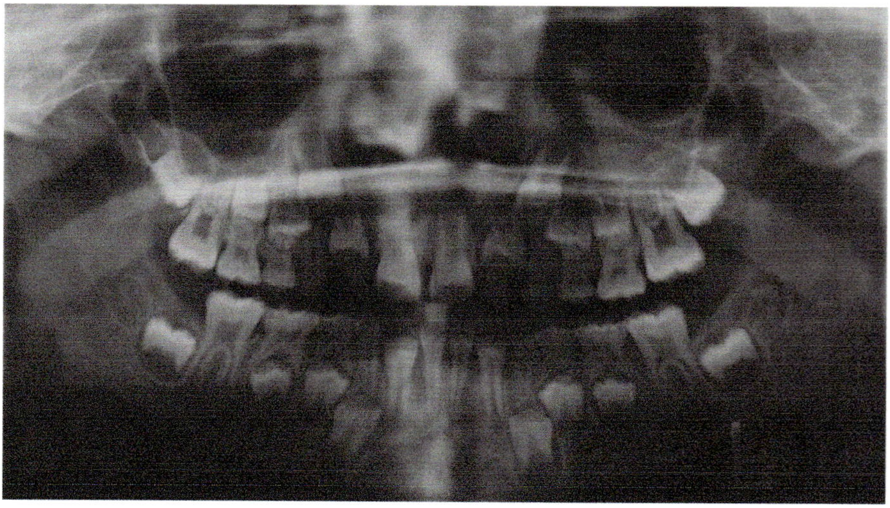

Fig. 3.10 Panoramic radiograph revealing moderate taurodontism of maxillary right and left permanent first molars

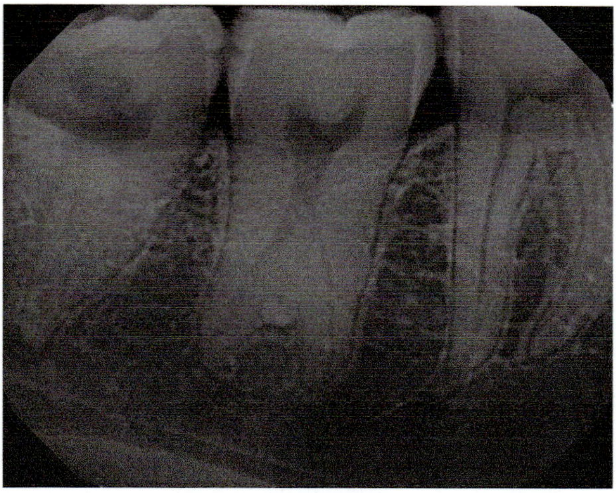

Fig. 3.11 Periapical radiograph revealing severe taurodontism of mandibular permanent first molar with enamel pearl in furcation (courtesy of Dr. William J DiZinno)

or plate and hypodontia [3]. Taurodontism may occur as an isolated trait or in multiple syndromes such as Klinefelter's, Down, Ellis–van Creveld, tricho–dento–osseous types I, II, and III, and Wolf–Hirschhorn. Enlarged pulp chambers may also occur in vitamin D-dependent rickets, hypophosphatasia, some cases of dentinogenesis imperfecta, shell teeth, regional odontodysplasia, and ectodermal dysplasia [3, 9].

3.5.2 Etiology

A failure or delay of invagination of Hertwig's epithelial root sheath has been suggested as a causative factor [9]. The delay results in a furcation closer to the apex [10]. Chromosomal abnormalities may interfere with the morphological development of the tooth [3]. Genetic predispositions include X-linked vitamin D-resistant rickets, X-chromosome aneuploidies and families with autosomal dominant amelogenesis imperfecta, X-linked recessive Lowe syndrome, and sex chromosomal aberrations (e.g., XXX, and XYY) [3, 9].

3.5.3 Treatment/Management

Routine restorative care is not affected since the pulp does not extend into the crown of the tooth. The unusual morphology of the pulp becomes significant if vital pulp therapy or endodontic therapy is necessary with the possible presence of supernumerary roots or canals. Magnification is recommended to facilitate locating, instrumenting, and obturating pulp canals. Risks of root resorption and decreased anchorage due to reduced surface area negatively impact orthodontic treatment and use as an abutment tooth. Post-placement is not advisable. On a positive note, significant periodontal destruction must occur before the bifurcation of a taurodont molar is involved [3]. Thinner and shorter root apices make extraction more difficult [10].

3.6 Mesiodens

3.6.1 Description

The mesiodens (plural mesiodentes) is the most common supernumerary tooth and is typically located between the maxillary central incisors in a palatal position with inverted orientation (Fig. 3.12). The most common complication is a midline diastema (Fig. 3.13) followed by delayed eruption or displacement of the adjacent incisors [11]. The shape may be turberculate, supplemental (tooth-like), or conical (Figs. 3.14 and 3.15). Conical is the most common morphology with a completely formed short root. Over-retention of a primary central incisor is a common clinical presentation (Fig. 3.16). A periapical radiograph may affirm a mesiodens as the causative circumstance (Fig. 3.17). Additional clinical presentations are delayed, ectopic eruption or impaction of a maxillary permanent incisor [12]. Arrested root development, dilaceration of developing roots, and bone deformities are also associated with a mesiodens. Scrutiny of upper occlusal, periapical, or panoramic radiograph may reveal an unsuspected mesiodens (Figs. 3.18 and 3.19). A mesiodens may not be as evident on a panoramic due to the lack of clarity in the midline area. Cone-beam computed tomography provides more definitive information prior to extraction. Mesiodentes often occur with cleft lip and palate, Gardner syndrome, and cleidocranial dysostosis [13].

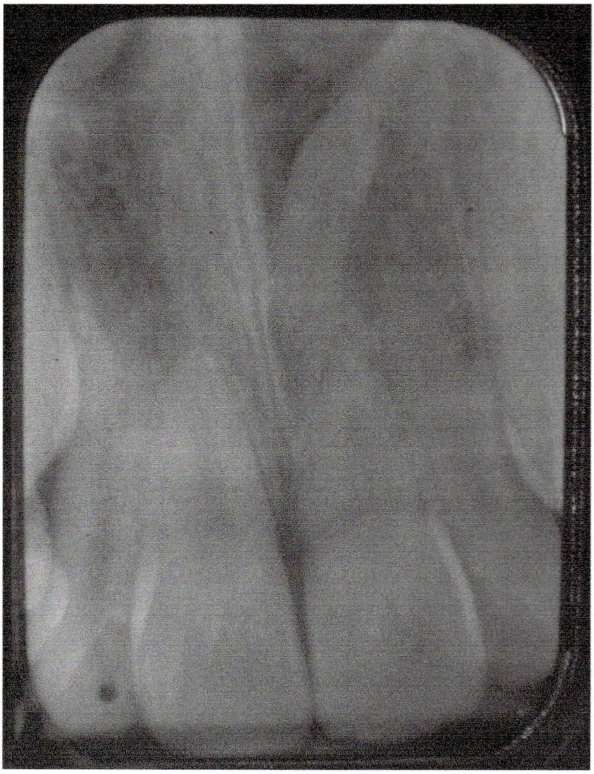

Fig. 3.12 Periapical radiograph revealing inverted mesiodens

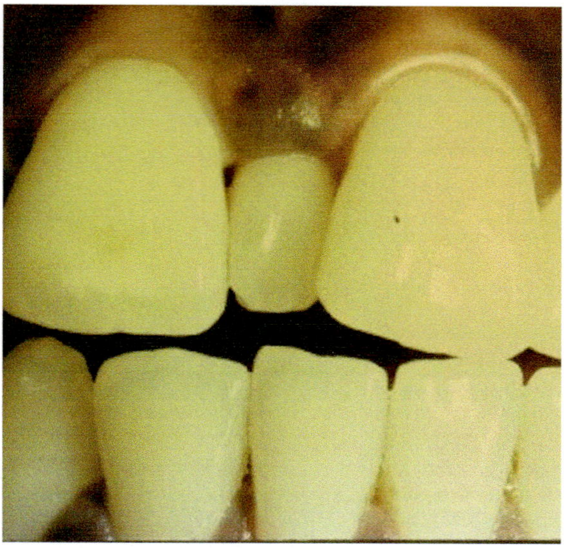

Fig. 3.13 Clinical photograph showing diastema with erupted mesiodens (courtesy of Dr. William J DiZinno)

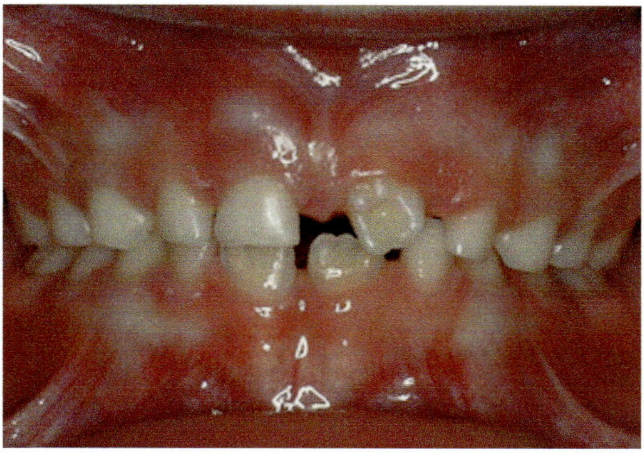

Fig. 3.14 Clinical photograph showing turberculate mesiodens

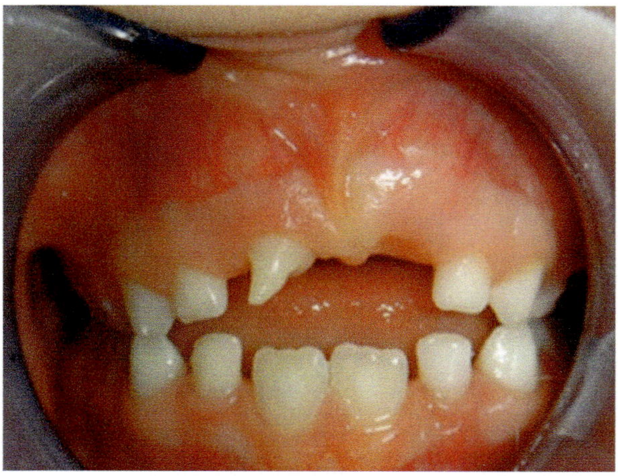

Fig. 3.15 Clinical photograph showing conical mesiodens

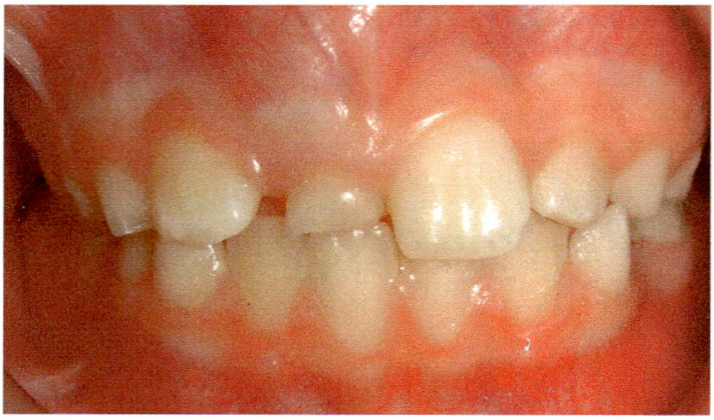

Fig. 3.16 Clinical photograph showing over-retained maxillary right primary central incisor due to mesiodens causing impaction of maxillary right permanent incisor

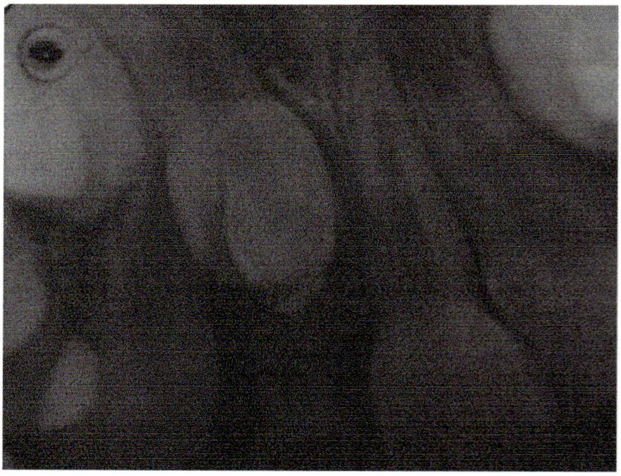

Fig. 3.17 Periapical radiograph revealing impaction of maxillary right permanent central incisor caused by mesiodens

3.6.2 Etiology

Causative factors include both environmental and genetic. Developmentally, mesiodens occurs in the dental lamina formation stage during induction and proliferation [9]. Local hyperactivity of the dental lamina has been proposed, along with both autosomal-dominant and autosomal-recessive genes. Skipped generations may occur. The incidence of occurrence is twofold between males and females, which supports an X-linked mode of inheritance [13].

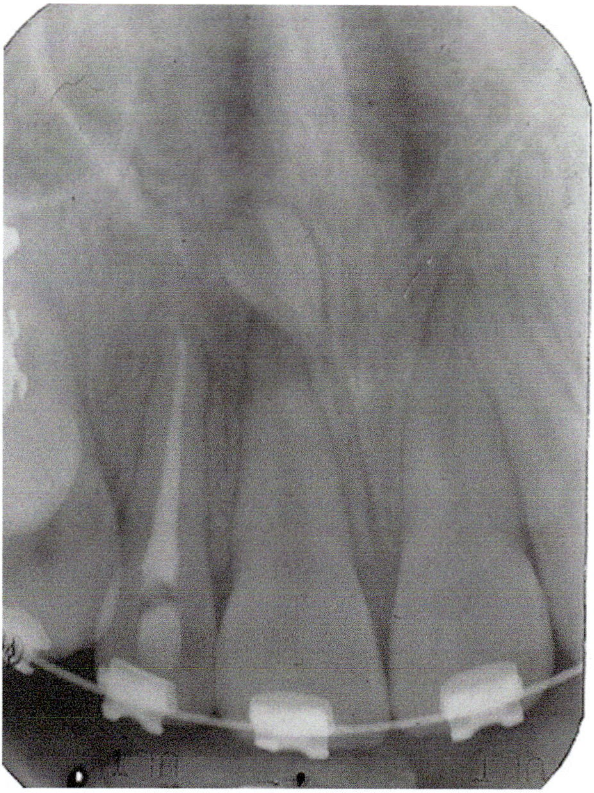

Fig. 3.18 Periapical radiograph revealing mesiodens

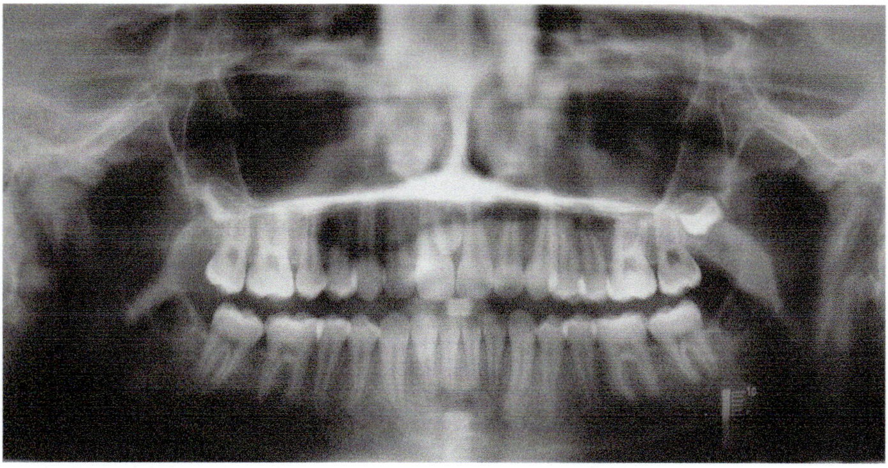

Fig. 3.19 Panoramic radiograph revealing mesiodens

3.6.3 Treatment/Management

Resorption of the roots of adjacent permanent incisors may occur; so following with periodic radiographs is advisable. If deemed necessary, surgical extraction of the mesiodens is the most common treatment. Extraction at 6–7 years of age has been recommended to avoid damage to the root of the developing incisor and minimize risk of developmental complications. Post-extraction, the permanent incisor erupts without further intervention in the majority of cases. If diagnosis is delayed until after complete root formation of the permanent central incisor, surgical exposure of the impacted incisor and orthodontic treatment for assisted eruption may be necessary. Delayed extraction of a mesiodens may also result in drifting of the maxillary permanent laterals into the space for the permanent incisor with a resulting midline shift and the need for orthodontic treatment to open the space. Conical mesiodentes with normal orientation, located above the apices of the developing permanent incisors, are an exception to early extraction [13, 14].

References

1. Liuk IW, Olive RJ, Griffin M et al (2013) Maxillary lateral incisor morphology and palatally displaced canines: a case-controlled cone-beam volumetric tomography study. Am J Orthod Dentofac Orthop 143:522–526
2. Kulshrestha R (2016) Interdisciplinary approach in the treatment of peg lateral incisors. J Orthod Endod 2:1
3. Neville BW, Damm DD, Allen CM, Chi AC (2016) Abnormalities of teeth. In: Oral and maxillofacial pathology, 4th edn. Elsevier, St. Louis, pp 80–82, 86–87
4. Saini TS, Kharat DU, Mokeem S (1990) Prevalence of shovel-shaped incisors in Saudi Arabian dental patients. Oral Surg Oral Med Oral Pathol 70(4):540–544
5. Kimura R, Yamaguchi T, Takeda M et al (2009) A common variation in EDAR is a genetic determinant of shovel-shaped incisors. Am J Hum Genet 85(4):528–535
6. Kirthiga M, Manju M, Praveen R, Umesh W (2015) Prevalence of aberrant dental morphological details in 6–10 year old school children in an Indian population. Contemp Clin Dent 6(Suppl 1):S175–S180
7. Nirmala SVSG, Challa R, Velpula L et al (2011) Unusual occurrence of accessory cusp in the maxillary second primary molar. Contemp Clin Dent 2(2):127–130
8. Ozcelik B, Atila B (2011) Bilateral palatal talon cusps on permanent maxillary lateral incisors: a case report. Eur J Dent 5(1):113–116
9. Cameron AC, Widmer RP (eds) (2008) Dental anomalies. In: Handbook of pediatric dentistry, 3rd edn. Mosby, London, pp 242–245
10. Klein U, Paimagham B, Blumhagen R et al (2017) Pyramidal and taurodont molars and their association with other tooth anomalies. Pediatr Dent 39(1):46–52
11. Jung Y-H, Kim J-Y, Cho B-H (2016) The effects of impacted premaxillary supernumerary teeth on permanent incisors. Imaging Sci Dent 46:251–258
12. Dongmei H, Li M, Wang Y (2017) Association between maxillary anterior supernumerary teeth and impacted incisors in the mixed dentition. J Am Dent Assoc 148:595–603
13. Soxman JA (2015) Diagnosis and management of mesiodentes. Gen Dent 63(5):18–19
14. Omer RS, Anthronappa RP, King NM (2010) Determination of the optimum time for surgical removal of unerupted anterior supernumerary teeth. Pediatr Dent 32(1):14–20

Anomalies of Tooth Number

4

4.1 Introduction

Hypodontia, which presents with agenesis of one or multiple teeth, occurs due to absence of appropriate dental lamina during tooth formation. Hyperdontia describes an increased number of teeth resulting from a disorder during the proliferation stage of tooth development. Both anomalies are the result of genetic influences and associated with multiple syndromes.

4.2 Hypodontia/Anodontia

A lack of the initiation stage of tooth development in the dental lamina formation stage of tooth development results in the absence of a single tooth or multiple teeth [1]. The most frequently missing teeth are the maxillary permanent lateral incisors, maxillary and mandibular second premolars, and/or third molars (Figs. 4.1, 4.2, and 4.3) [2]. Different terms are used to describe the variations in number of teeth. Hypodontia is the absence of one or more teeth. Oligodontia is a subdivision of hypodontia and denotes lack of development of six or more teeth, not including third molars (Fig. 4.4). Anodontia describes the absence of tooth formation [3].

4.2.1 Description

Hypodontia is one of the most commonly occurring developmental anomalies. Prevalence is 3–10% in the permanent dentition excluding third molars with a 1.5:1 predilection in females versus males. Permanent maxillary central incisors, mandibular first molars, and canines are least often missing. Ethnic variations occur with mandibular central incisors most often missing in Chinese populations.

J. A. Soxman et al., *Anomalies of the Developing Dentition*,
https://doi.org/10.1007/978-3-030-03164-0_4

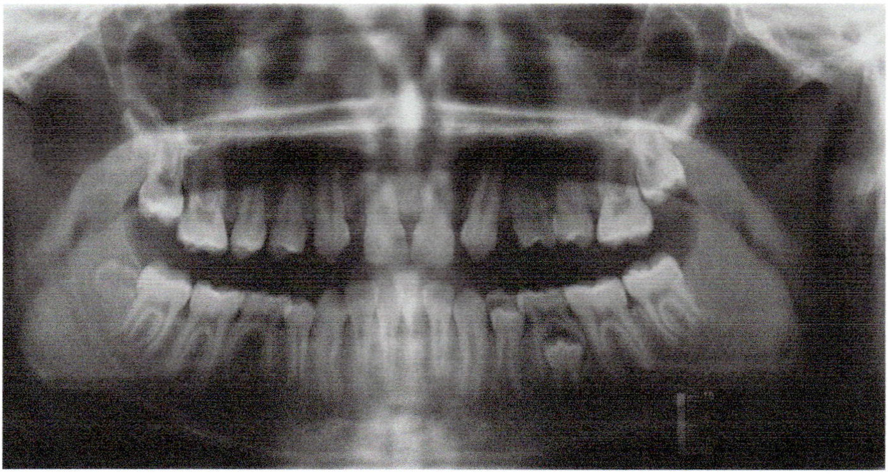

Fig. 4.1 Panoramic radiograph revealing the absence of maxillary right and left permanent lateral incisors, mandibular right second premolar, and mandibular left third molar

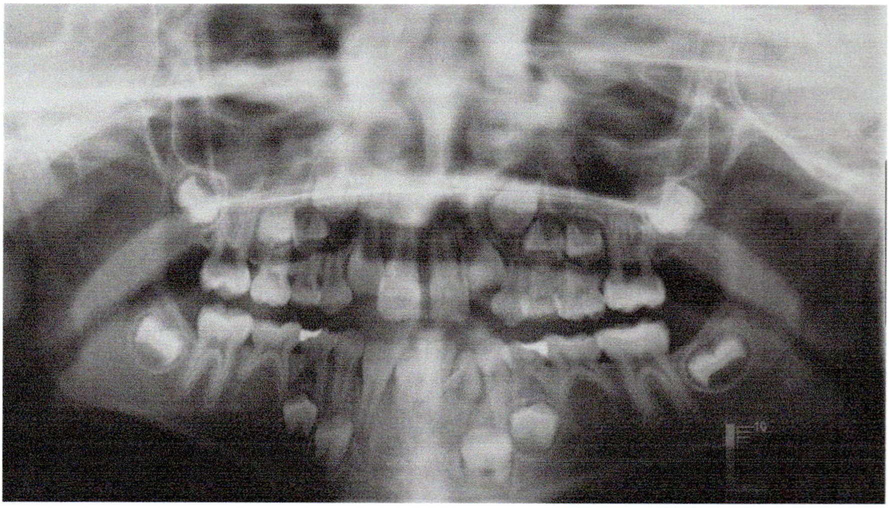

Fig. 4.2 Panoramic radiograph revealing the absence of mandibular right and left second premolars

American blacks have significantly lower incidence of missing teeth, and 80% of Caucasians are congenitally missing only one or two teeth. Associated with missing permanent teeth are diminished alveolar bone development, anterior malocclusion, over-retention of primary teeth, and microdontia [3]. A submerged primary molar may signal a missing premolar (Figs. 4.5 and 4.6). Absence of a primary tooth is strongly associated with the absence of its successor.

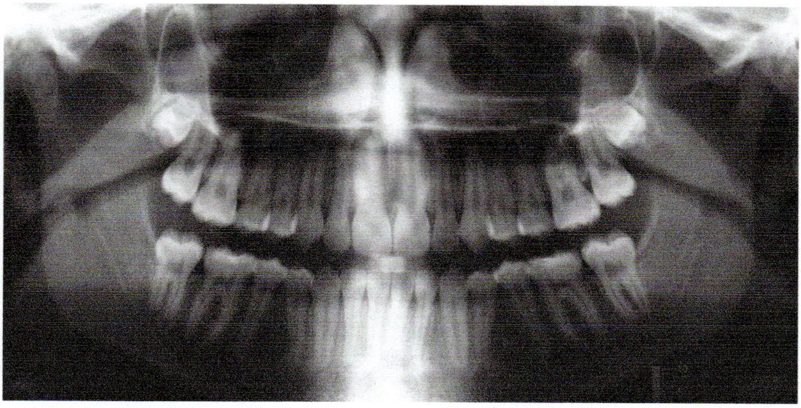

Fig. 4.3 Panoramic radiograph revealing the absence of mandibular right and left third molars

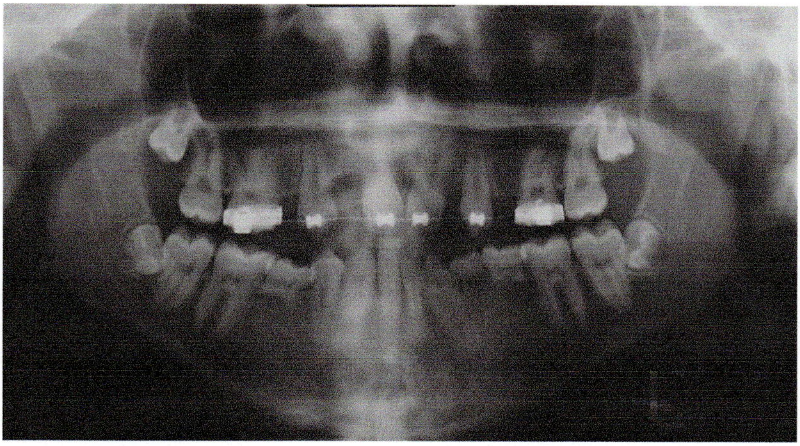

Fig. 4.4 Panoramic radiograph revealing oligodontia with agenesis of development of more than six permanent teeth

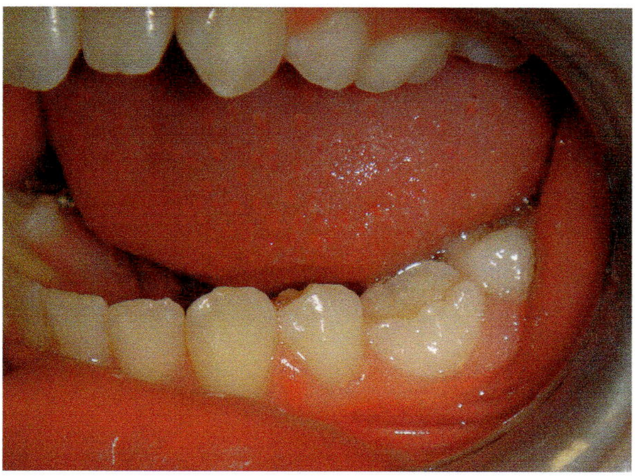

Fig. 4.5 Clinical photograph showing submerged mandibular second primary molar

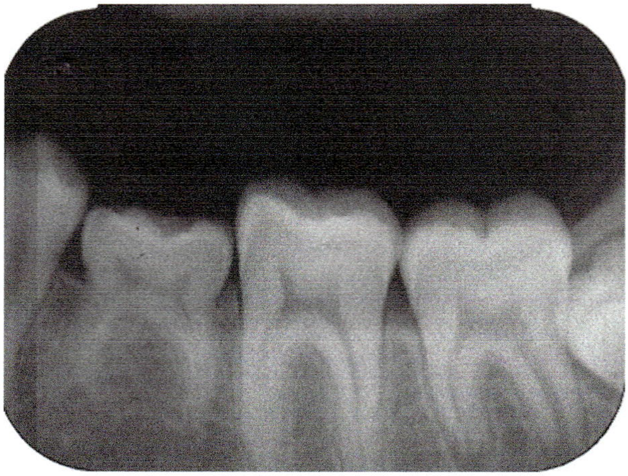

Fig. 4.6 Periapical radiograph revealing submerged mandibular second primary molar with agenesis of second premolar

4.2.2 Etiology

Genetics plays a fundamental role in the etiology of tooth agenesis with more than 200 genes involved [3]. Genetic mutations are often associated with hypodontia. Mutation of the AXIN2 gene is inherited as an autosomal dominant disorder. The teeth most commonly missing are the second and third permanent molars, second premolars, maxillary lateral incisors, and the mandibular incisors. With this presentation, questioning family medical history is strongly suggested, since a known association exists with adenomatous polyps and colorectal cancer. Mutation of the PAX9 gene results in an autosomal dominant pattern of missing teeth that most often affects permanent molars. Another autosomal dominant trait inherited with mutation of the MSX1 gene typically presents with congenitally missing posterior teeth. The second premolars and third molars are most commonly missing, but the maxillary first premolars and lateral incisors are also missing in more severe cases. Inheritance may also be autosomal recessive or X-linked with considerable variation in expression and penetrance [4].

More than 50 syndromes exhibit hypodontia as a major feature. These include ectodermal dysplasia (Fig. 4.7), Down syndrome, chondroectodermal dysplasia, Rieger syndrome, Craniosynostosis syndrome, incontinentia pigmenti, oro-facial-digital syndrome, Williams' syndrome, and dentoalveolar clefting with disruption of the dental lamina at that site (Cameron and Widmer). Multiple dental anomalies may signal a recommendation for genetic counseling as seen with radiographic evidence in a male with XYY syndrome (Fig. 4.8).

Agenesis of maxillary lateral incisors is often accompanied by other dental anomalies that appear in the same patient. These anomalies include delayed dental development, microdontia of the contralateral maxillary lateral incisor, palatal displacement of maxillary canines, and distal angulation of mandibular second premolars. Speculation is that genetic mutations may be responsible for a series of diverse phenotypic expressions [5, 6].

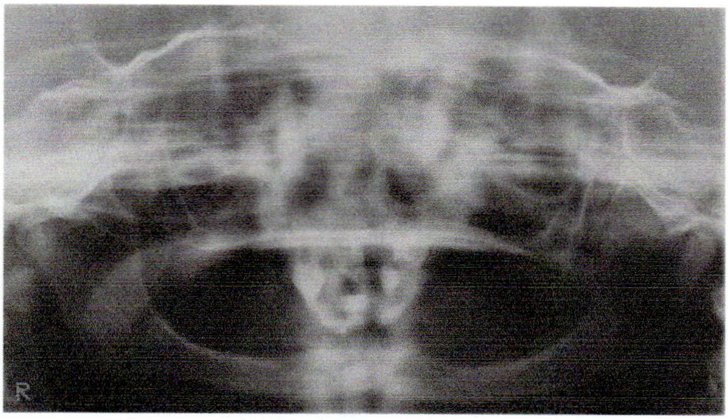

Fig. 4.7 Panoramic radiograph revealing agenesis of multiple teeth with ectodermal dysplasia

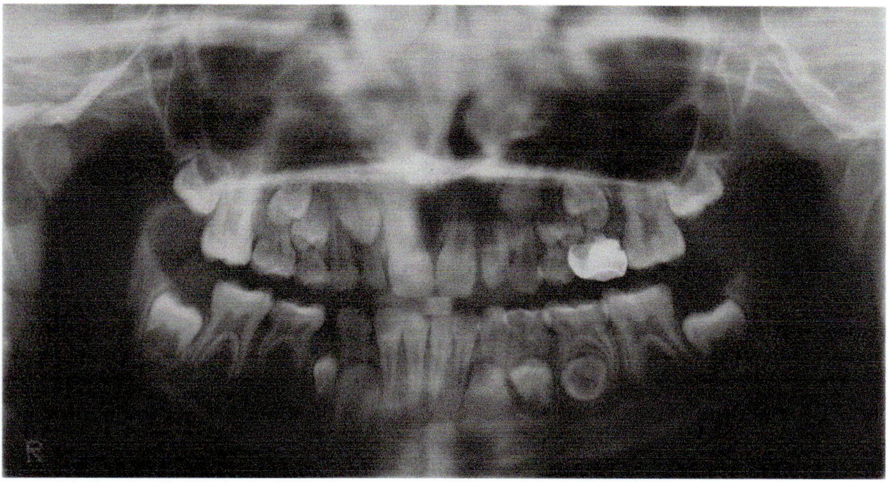

Fig. 4.8 Panoramic radiograph revealing multiple anomalies with XYY syndrome

Teeth missing unilaterally in a single or both quadrants may be the result of radiation to the face at a young age. The developing permanent tooth is very sensitive to radiation. Even with low dosage, radiation may destroy the tooth buds or cause stunting if partial calcification has already occurred [7, 8].

4.2.3 Treatment/Management

The first evidence of a missing permanent tooth may be an over-retained or submerged primary tooth, confirmed with radiographic examination. First and second premolars begin calcification between 18–24 months and 24–30 months of age, respectively. Third molars begin calcification at 7–9 years of age in the maxilla and 8–10 years of age in the mandible [9]. Absence of formation prior to that time with average ages for development of the permanent dentition should not be mistaken for agenesis.

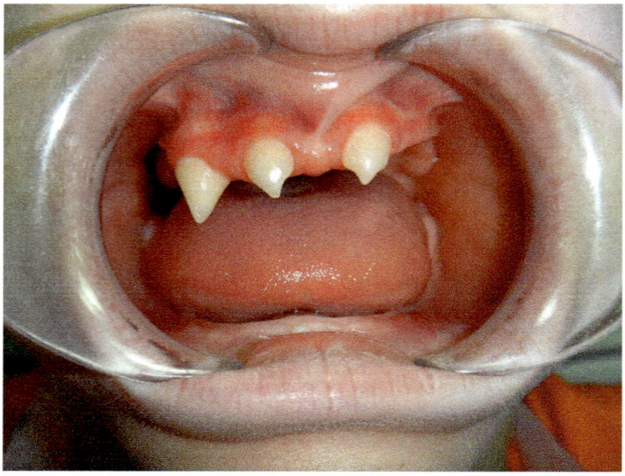

Fig. 4.9 Clinical photograph showing conical anterior teeth as seen in ectodermal dysplasia

To determine short- and long-term treatment goals and reduce negative effect on craniofacial growth, early collaboration among dental specialists is advised. Esthetics, social considerations, function, stable occlusion, and maintenance of space and vertical dimension are considerations in a timely treatment plan that includes current and future needs. Additionally, finances, compliance, and oral and systemic health will influence care.

Ectodermal dysplasia requires early intervention beginning in the primary dentition. If behavior permits, the conical anterior teeth (Fig. 4.9) can be reshaped with composite for a more esthetic appearance. Later a partial denture, conventional or overdenture, primarily for esthetics and vertical dimension, can be fabricated. Because alveolar bone does not develop in the absence of teeth, retention of a denture may be significantly compromised. Dentures can be relined or re-fabricated to accommodate growth and retention. Composite resin or orthodontic buttons can be bonded to the teeth to aid in retention of the denture or for removable appliance clasps. Conical teeth may be restored with composite resin buildup or composite resin crowns. Composite veneers, crowns, and laboratory-fabricated bridges are additional treatment options. Although the recommendation is to await completion of craniofacial growth prior to placing implants, ectodermal dysplasia may be an appropriate circumstance for earlier implant placement. Research indicates that implants placed in the canine area of the mandible around 8–10 years of age will aid in lower denture retention. At this time, maximal transverse growth of the mandible is complete [1].

Intervention for space closure or esthetics may not be necessary with agenesis of a mandibular incisor (Fig. 4.10). Maxillary and mandibular midlines may not be aligned, but this typically is of no concern with function or esthetics.

Early intervention with orthodontic collaboration to determine the appropriate treatment course for primary molars without a permanent successor is advised. Primary teeth without permanent successors may be maintained to aid in alveolar ridge preservation for a future implant and prosthetic crown. Bone levels between

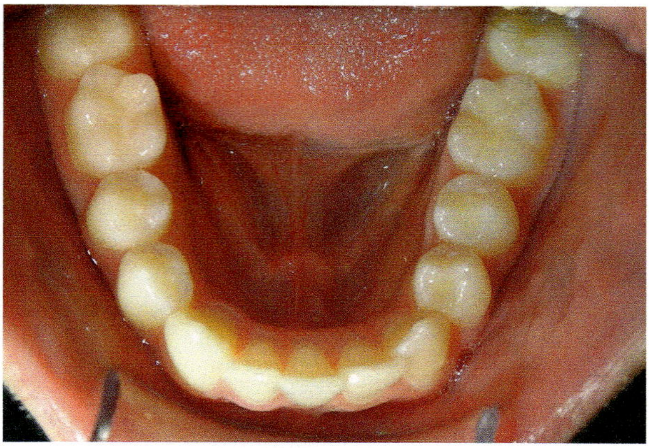

Fig. 4.10 Clinical photograph showing agenesis of mandibular incisor requiring no intervention

the submerged primary molar and adjacent teeth should be monitored with periapical radiographs to assure continued horizontal bone level without vertical bone loss. If a vertical defect occurs, due to delaying extraction, additional treatment costs will likely be incurred with bone grafting for an osseo-integrated implant [10]. Reduction of the mesiodistal width of the primary molar with disking can be performed to optimize the space for a future implant and prosthetic crown. Primary molars are typically 1–2 mm wider than their successors [4]. The average width of a mandibular second premolar is 7.5 mm [11]. A guideline to determine mesiodistal width reduction is measuring the width of the primary molar at the cementoenamel junction on a bitewing or periapical radiograph. Comparison to the contralateral premolar can also be used to determine mesiodistal width. If the primary molar is submerged, adding composite resin to the occlusal surface will maintain a level occlusal plane and prevent super-eruption of the opposing tooth in the upper arch. A zirconia primary molar crown or composite resin crown (Fig. 4.11) are good options for esthetics, providing augmented occlusal height, and corrected mesiodistal width for future implant [12]. A stainless steel crown is another option. After eruption of the permanent first molar, another option may be extraction of the primary molar, followed by space maintenance and/or orthodontic space closure [1]. If orthodontic space closure is not possible, a space maintainer can maintain the space until an osseo-integrated implant is performed when facial growth is complete. Primary molars without a permanent successor may be retained for many years. With no evidence of ankylosis, natural exfoliation may be permitted [10, 12].

Multiple approaches are possible for treatment of missing permanent lateral incisors. Removable appliances, canine substitution with space closure, resin-bonded fixed partial dentures (FPD), conventional full-coverage FPD, and osseo-integrated implants are treatment alternatives. If acceptable esthetics can be achieved with orthodontic-assisted space closure, the primary lateral incisor may substitute for the missing permanent lateral incisor (Fig. 4.12). As with missing mandibular second premolars, interdisciplinary treatment is necessary. The preferred treatment choice will be based on various factors. Kokich et al. divide restorative treatment into two

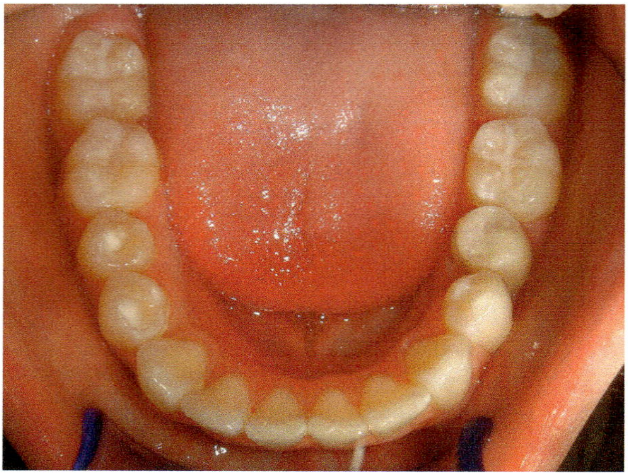

Fig. 4.11 Clinical photograph showing composite resin restoration to reshape submerged mandibular left second primary molar with augmented occlusal height and mesiodistal reduction to match contralateral premolar

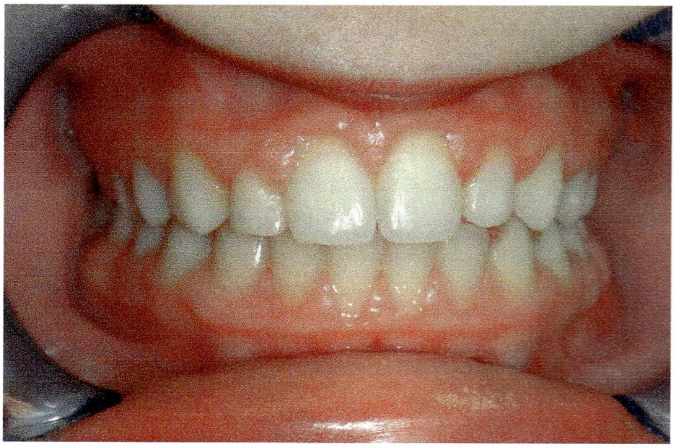

Fig. 4.12 Clinical photograph showing maxillary right primary lateral incisor substituting for permanent lateral incisor

categories: single-tooth implant and tooth-supported restoration. A resin-bonded FPD, a cantilevered FPD, and full-coverage FPD are three options for a tooth-supported restoration. Conservation of tooth structure is the most important factor in treatment choice, meeting the esthetic and functional criteria. Collaboration with an orthodontist is usually required to position the adjacent teeth with coronal and apical spacing for the selected restorative plan.

Before facial growth is complete, interim tooth replacement is necessary. A removable appliance with a prosthetic incisor provides improved esthetics prior to orthodontic intervention.

A removable appliance is not recommended for retention post-orthodontic treatment, because the roots of the central incisors and canines may converge toward each other, complicating or negating future implant placement. Fixed retainers such as a bonded lingual wire with a prosthetic incisor or a laboratory-fabricated resin-bonded bridge (Fig. 4.13) or porcelain fused to metal bridge (Figs. 4.14 and 4.15) are preferred methods for retention prior to completion of facial growth [13].

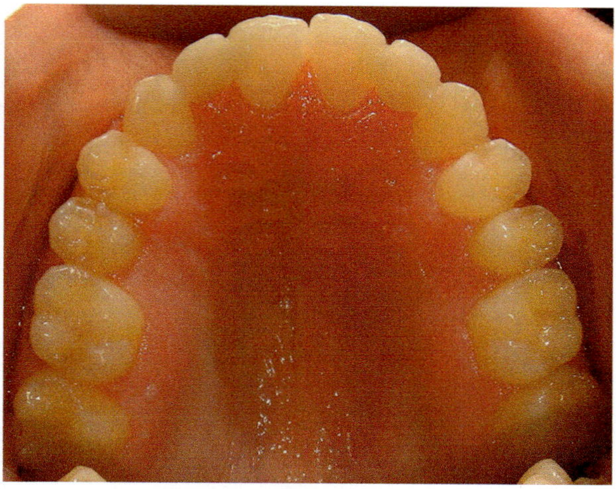

Fig. 4.13 Clinical photograph showing occlusal view of laboratory-fabricated resin-bonded bridge to replace missing maxillary left permanent lateral incisor

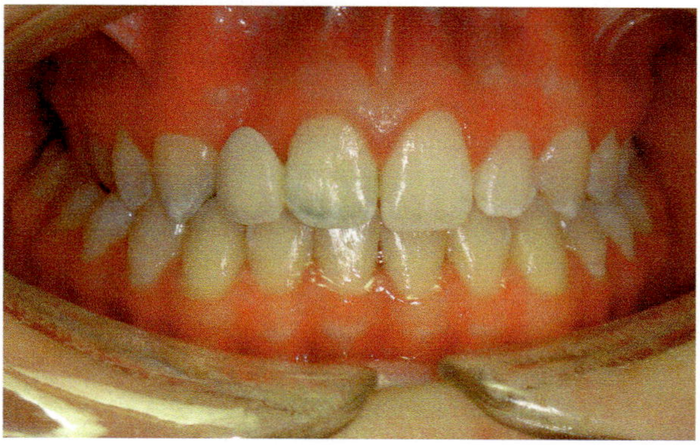

Fig. 4.14 Clinical photograph showing facial view of Maryland bridge to replace missing maxillary right permanent lateral incisor

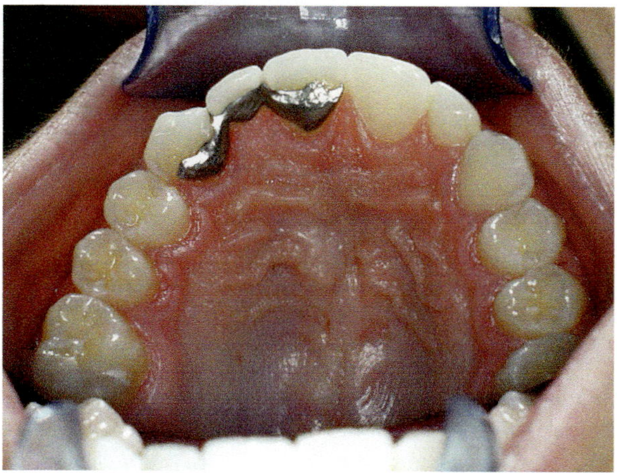

Fig. 4.15 Clinical photograph showing occlusal view of Maryland bridge to replace missing maxillary permanent lateral incisor

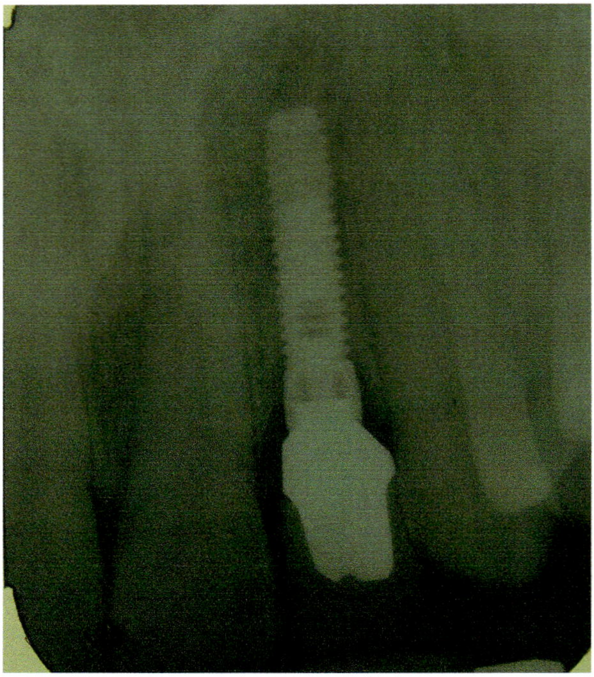

Fig. 4.16 Periapical radiograph showing implant for agenesis of maxillary left permanent lateral incisor

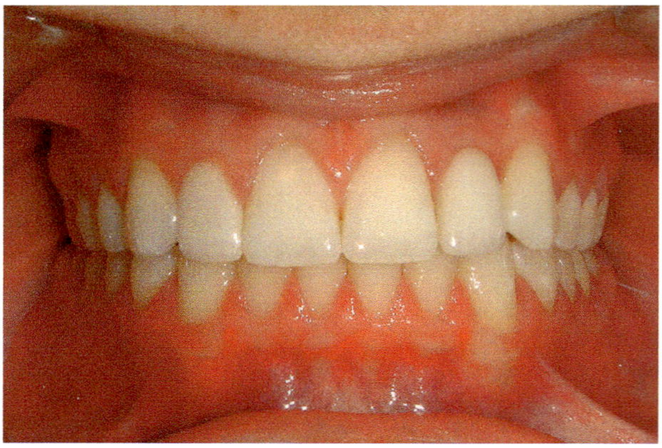

Fig. 4.17 Clinical photograph showing facial view of prosthetic crown for agenesis of maxillary left permanent lateral incisor

After growth is complete, the single-tooth implant is the favored choice for replacement of the missing incisor (Figs. 4.16 and 4.17). Facial growth is the main factor in determining time for implant placement. With increase in the vertical height of the rami, the dentition must erupt to remain in occlusion. Because implants do not erupt, placement of an implant prior to completion of facial growth may result in not only occlusal but periodontal and esthetic complications. Hand-wrist radiographs do not accurately predict the cessation of facial growth. The most reliable method to show growth with increase in vertical facial height is superimposing

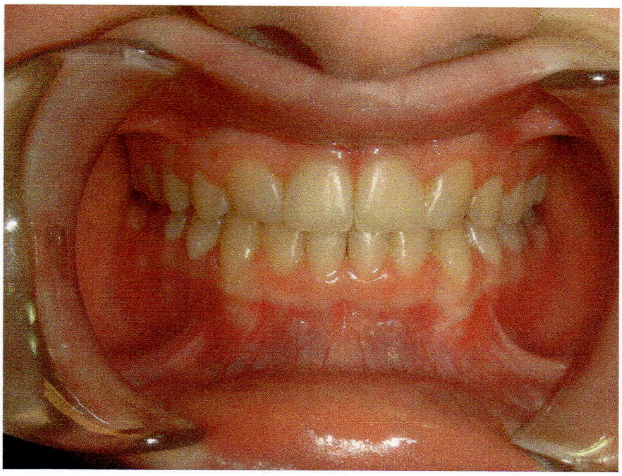

Fig. 4.18 Clinical photograph showing facial view of canine substitution after orthodontic repositioning and reshaping maxillary right and left permanent canines

serial cephalometric radiographs, taken 6 months to 1 year apart. Implants can be performed after growth cessation, about 20–21 years of age in males and 16–17 years of age in females [13].

An implant may not be an option due to the patient's lack of desire to undergo orthodontic treatment or necessary ridge augmentation, or a site for ideal implant placement is not achievable. When considering the least invasive tooth replacement, the resin-bonded FPD is the treatment choice; since adjacent teeth are not touched. However, debonding is a common cause of failure, associated with deep bite and proclined teeth. The most ideal circumstance for use of a resin-bonded FPD is shallow over-bite, nonmobile, upright abutments, and a patient who does not brux. The cantilevered FPD provides more predictability, but all contacts in excursive movements must be eliminated. Since the conventional full-coverage FPD is the most invasive, it is used only when replacing an existing full-coverage bridge or when adjacent teeth are carious or fractured.

Canine substitution (Figs. 4.18 and 4.19) is another alternative for management of missing maxillary lateral incisors, which also requires interdisciplinary involvement of the general dentist or prosthodontist and the orthodontist. Space closure is achieved with orthodontic movement of the canine(s) into the space. Management of the difference in size, shape, color, root volume, and height of the gingival margin of the canine presents challenges. The canine is longer and wider mesiodistally and buccolingually, and more saturated with color. In addition, the first premolar may be shorter and narrower than the contralateral canine, requiring additional intervention with veneers or extraction. The canine(s) are reshaped, bleached, or restored with veneers or composite to achieve an esthetic result. The alveolar bone height in the area of mesial tooth movement is maintained, and final results can be achieved in early adolescence [14].

A systematic review of studies that compared and evaluated functional, periodontal, and esthetic outcomes of prosthetic treatment versus canine substitution found orthodontic space closure to be preferable to prosthetic replacement [15].

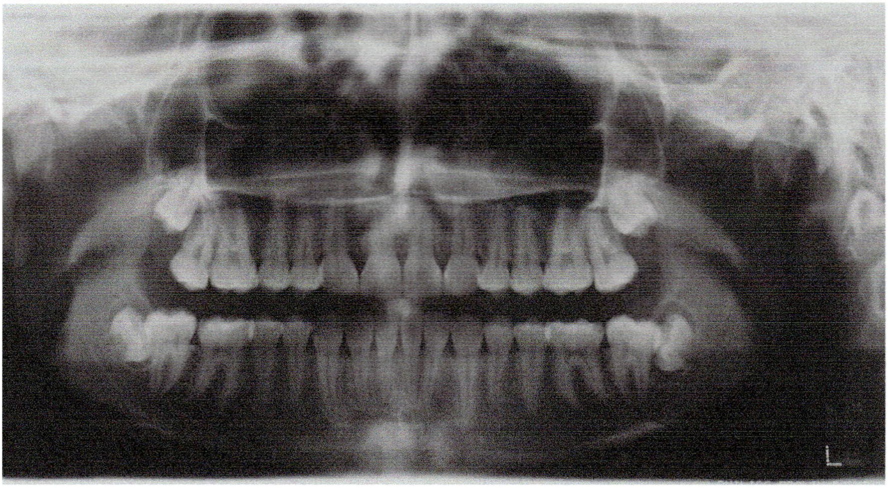

Fig. 4.19 Panoramic radiograph revealing orthodontically repositioned maxillary right and left permanent canines into space for missing right and left permanent lateral incisors

4.3 Hyperdontia/Supernumerary Teeth

This anomaly occurs in the dental lamina formation stage during induction and proliferation [1]. Respectively, prevalence is maxillary anterior, maxillary and mandibular fourth molars (Fig. 4.20), premolars, canines, and lateral incisors. Supernumerary teeth may also occur in areas of the oral cavity other than the alveolar ridges such as soft palate, maxillary sinus, nasal cavity, between the orbit and brain, and the sphenomaxillary fissure [3].

4.3.1 Description

As with hypodontia, ethnic variations occur with supernumerary teeth. Prevalence in Caucasians varies from 0.1% to 3.8% with a slightly higher occurrence in Asians. American blacks show increased frequency up to nine times higher than whites. In terms of gender, males show a two-to-one predominance over females. Single-tooth hyperdontia occurs in 76–86% of cases, primarily in the permanent dentition with 95% in the maxillary arch, predominately in the anterior. The incidence of two supernumerary teeth ranges from 12% to 23% and three or more occur in <1%.

Supernumerary teeth are classified by form and location. Mesiodens (Chap. 3) typically occur in the maxillary incisor area. These teeth are termed either supplemental or rudimentary. Supplemental teeth are normal in shape and size, whereas rudimentary teeth are smaller in size with abnormal shape. Rudimentary teeth are further classified as peg-shaped/conical, barrel-shaped/tuberculate in the anterior with one or more cusps, and small premolar or molar-like in shape/molariform.

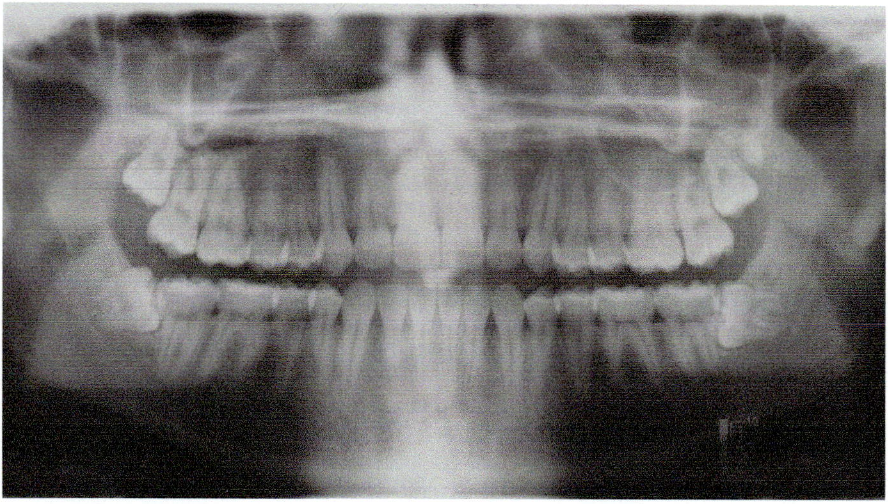

Fig. 4.20 Panoramic radiograph revealing maxillary left fourth molar

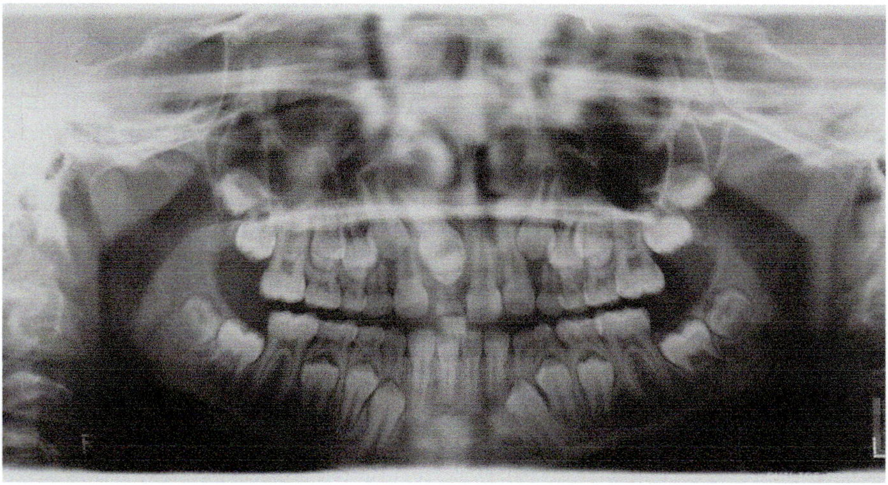

Fig. 4.21 Panoramic radiograph revealing failed eruption of maxillary right permanent central incisor caused by supernumerary incisor

Conical mesiodens erupt spontaneously. Tuberculate shaped, which occur less frequently, typically do not erupt [3]. A fourth molar is termed a distomolar or distodens, and a supernumerary tooth located in the posterior that is buccal or lingual to a molar is termed paramolar [3].

Failed or delayed eruption of a permanent tooth (Fig. 4.21), a large diastema, or malalignment of an incisor may be clinical ramifications of a supernumerary.

4.3.2 Etiology

Supernumerary teeth occur as the result of budding of the dental lamina sporadically or via inheritance. Cleidocranial dysplasia, a condition that includes multiple supernumerary teeth, is inherited via an autosomal dominant mode and includes a high frequency of genetic mutations [1].

4.3.3 Treatment/Management

An upper occlusal or periapical radiograph may be more diagnostic than a panoramic for diagnosing anterior supernumerary teeth, because the clarity of a panoramic in the anterior often is poor. Periapical radiographs with shift shots can be used to determine the location of an anterior supernumerary, but a vertex occlusal more accurately identifies the anteroposterior position of the tooth. Digital imaging with cone beam tomography provides high-definition and three-dimensional imaging with less radiation exposure than traditional computer tomography [1]. Impaction of maxillary incisors is associated with supernumerary teeth in the anterior segment of the maxilla [16]. Timely extraction of a supernumerary is recommended in the mixed dentition to avoid clinical complications of adjacent teeth such as delayed eruption, root resorption, displacement due to crowding, dilaceration, eruption into the nasal cavity, malocclusion, and large diastema. These complications occur more often in the anterior than the posterior. Eruption of the permanent tooth occurs in the majority of cases after extraction of the supernumerary. However, permanent teeth with closed apices may require surgical exposure with orthodontic assistance for eruption [3]. Tuberculate mesiodens have an increased incidence of non-eruption, resulting in crowding, displacement, or rotations of adjacent teeth requiring orthodontic intervention [17, 18].

References

1. Cameron AC, Widmer RP (eds) (2008) Dental anomalies. In: Handbook of pediatric dentistry, 3rd edn. Mosby, London, pp 219–231
2. Kumar GS (2011) In: Bhaskar SN (ed) Orban's oral histology and embryology. Elsevier, New Delhi, p 46
3. Neville BW, Damm DD, Allen CM, Chi AC (2016) Abnormalities of teeth. In: Oral and maxillofacial pathology, 4th edn. Elsevier, St. Louis, pp 70–76
4. Cooper LF (2015) Treatment of nonsyndromic anomalies of tooth number. In: Wright T (ed) Craniofacial and dental developmental defects: diagnosis and management. Springer, Basel, pp 49–61
5. Garib DG, Alencar BM, Lauris JRP et al (2010) Agenesis of maxillary lateral incisors and associated dental anomalies. Am J Orthod Dentofac Orthop 137:732.e1–732.e6
6. Liuk IW, Olive RJ, Griffin M et al (2013) Maxillary lateral incisor morphology and palatally displaced canines: a case-controlled cone-beam volumetric tomography study. Am J Orthod Dentofac Orthop 143:522–526

7. Javed F, Utreja A, Correa FOB et al (2012) Oral health status in children with acute lymphoblastic leukemia. Crit Rev Oncol Hematol 83:303–309
8. Shafer WG, Hine MK, Levy BM (1974) Developmental disturbances of oral and para oral structures. In: A textbook of oral pathology, 3rd edn. W. B. Saunders, Philadelphia, p 42
9. American Academy of Pediatric Dentistry (2017) Dental growth and development. Pediatr Dent 39(6):456
10. Sabri R (2004) Management of congenitally missing second premolars with orthodontics and single tooth implants. Am J Orthod Dentofac Orthop 125:634–642
11. Kokich VG, Kokich VO (2006) Congenitally missing mandibular second premolars: clinical options. Am J Orthod Dentofac Orthop 130:437–444
12. Soxman JA (2015) Infraocclusion of mandibular primary molars. In: Soxman JA (ed) Handbook of clinical techniques in pediatric dentistry. Wiley, Ames, p 129
13. Kokich VO, Kinzer GA, Janakievski J (2011) Congenitally missing maxillary lateral incisors: restorative replacement. Am J Orthod Dentofac Orthop 139:435–445
14. Zachrisson BU, Rosa M, Toreskog S (2011) Congenitally missing maxillary lateral incisors: canine substitution. Am J Orthod Dentofac Orthop 139:434–445
15. Silveira GS, de Almeida NV, Pereira DMT et al (2016) Prosthetic replacement vs space closure for maxillary lateral incisor agenesis: a systematic review. Am J Orthod Dentofac Orthop 150:228–237
16. Dongmei H, Li M, Wang Y (2017) Association between maxillary anterior supernumerary teeth and impacted incisors in the mixed dentition. J Am Dent Assoc 148:595–603
17. Eigbobo JO, Osagbemiro BB (2011) Bilateral tuberculate supernumerary teeth. Clin Pract 1(2):e30
18. Jung Y-H, Kim J-Y, Cho B-H (2016) The effects of impacted premaxillary supernumerary teeth on permanent incisors. Imaging Sci Dent 46:251–258

Anomalies of Tooth Eruption

5

5.1 Introduction

Numerous factors or theories have been used to describe the cause for abnormal eruption of teeth. Whether the tooth prematurely erupts or has an altered path of eruption, the actual cause is not precise. Position of the tooth germ, systemic conditions or syndromes, genetics, and other unknown factors have often been cited as reasons for eruptive anomalies. Treatment/management often requires an in depth knowledge of the growth and development of the child. Treatment success is dependent upon the proper timing for interceptive types of treatments.

5.2 Natal/Neonatal Teeth

5.2.1 Description

Natal and Neonatal teeth describe conditions where primary teeth erupt early with the former being present at birth and the later erupting within the first 30 days of life [1]. The majority of natal or neonatal teeth are of the normal primary dentition (approximately 90%), while the remainder are supernumerary teeth (Fig. 5.1) [2]. According to a study performed by Wang et al., the ratio of natal to neonatal teeth was approximately 3:1, with more females affected than males. The primary mandibular central incisors are affected 85% of the time followed by the maxillary centrals at 11%, the mandibular canines/molars at 3% and the maxillary canines/molars at 1% [1].

Clinical appearance of natal and neonatal teeth can vary with most having a hypoplastic layer of enamel with varying degrees of severity, the absence of root formation, lack of ample and vascularized pulp, irregular dentin formation and lack of cementum formation [3]. Clinically, the teeth may be of normal size and shape or have a more conical appearance and color that is an opaque yellowish-brown [3]. Due to the lack of root support, most natal and neonatal teeth are mobile and pose an aspiration risk [2].

J. A. Soxman et al., *Anomalies of the Developing Dentition*,
https://doi.org/10.1007/978-3-030-03164-0_5

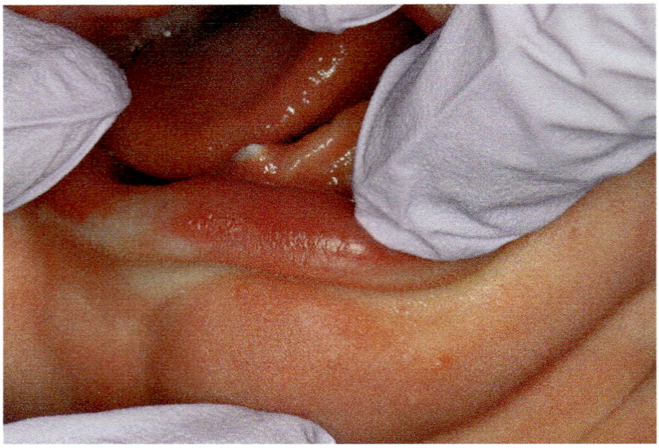

Fig. 5.1 Clinical photograph showing a natal tooth. (Courtesy of Dr. Tiffany Williams)

It is important to obtain a radiograph to assess root development and to verify whether the tooth is of the primary complement or a supernumerary tooth [3].

5.2.2 Etiology

The presence of natal and neonatal teeth is most likely due to an imbalance in the chronologic biology of unknown cause. Contributing factors include the superficial position of the tooth germ, infection, malnutrition/hypovitaminosis, fever, hormonal influences, hereditary influences and osteoblastic activity (remodeling) within the tooth germ [3]. Natal teeth may be associated with some syndromes such as Hallerman-Streiff, Ellis-Van Creveld, craniofacial dysostosis, multiple steacystoma, congenital pachyonychia, Sotos Syndrome and Rubenstein-Taybi Syndrome [3, 4]. There is a high prevalence of natal/neonatal teeth occurring in patients with cleft lip and palate (Fig. 5.2) [1] with the prevalence in one study occurring in 2% of patients with complete unilateral cleft lip and palate and 10% occurring in patients with complete bilateral cleft lip and palate [2].

Problems that can occur with natal/neonatal teeth include discomfort due to movement of the teeth resulting in a refusal to feed, sharp incisal edges that cause ulceration of the ventral surface of the tongue (Riga-Fede disease) and aspiration/swallowing risk during feeding [2]. According to Buchanan and Jenkins, 67% of natal and neonatal teeth will exfoliate prematurely however; only 38% exfoliate within the first year of life. Some natal teeth that have slight mobility and will often stabilize [5].

5.2.3 Treatment/Management

Treatment for natal/neonatal teeth that pose an irritation risk (Fig. 5.3) include smoothing off the incisal edge with a sandpaper disc or covering the incisal edge with composite; however the latter is more of a challenge due to difficulty in isolation and bonding to the hypoplastic enamel surface [5]. Treatment for extremely loose natal/ neonatal teeth is extraction however; extraction should not occur before the child is

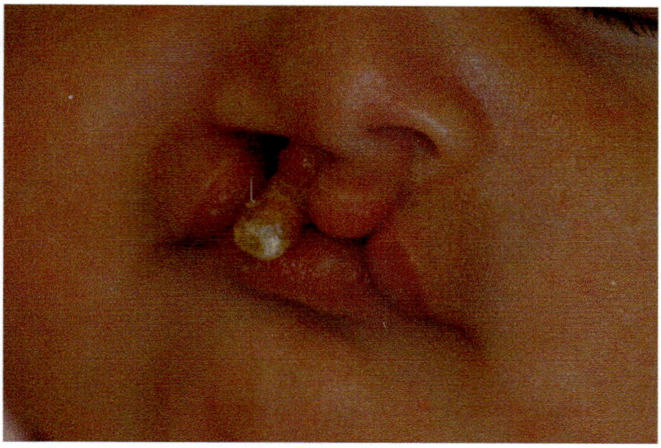

Fig. 5.2 Clinical photograph showing natal tooth in a patient with cleft lip and palate

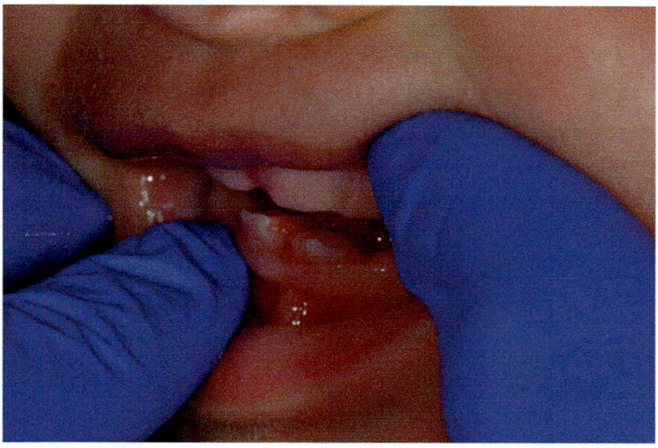

Fig. 5.3 Clinical photograph showing a natal tooth with sharp incisal edge. (Courtesy of Dr. Tiffany Williams)

10 days old. The 10-day wait period is necessary for the production of Vitamin K, which is essential for the production of prothrombin in the liver and important for clot formation [3]. In addition, when extracting these teeth, one should carefully curette out the socket to remove the remaining dental papilla; this may require the use of local anesthetic. During an extraction, when removal of only the external hard tissue occurs, it can result in leaving the internal dental papilla that continues to develop. This can also occur if the tooth exfoliates naturally or if the parent removes the crown with their finger, leaving behind the underlying dental papilla [6].

5.3 Ankylosis/Deep Submersion of Primary Molars

5.3.1 Description

Ankylosis describes an anatomical fusion between the cementum of the tooth root and the surrounding bone making it appear as if the affected tooth is sinking when in reality, the rest of the dentition continues to develop around a tooth that is anchored to the alveolar bone (Fig. 5.4) [7]. There are various terms used to

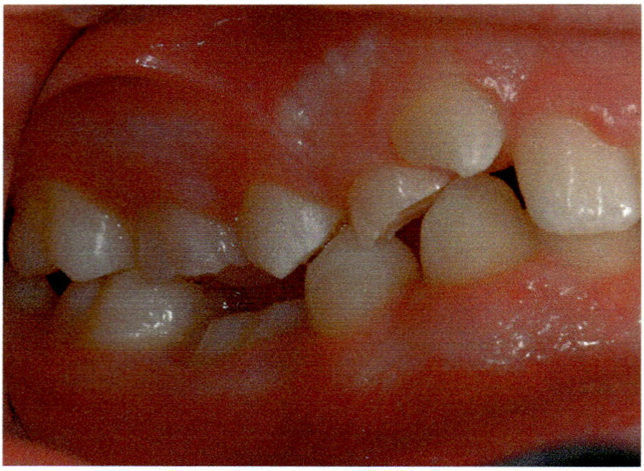

Fig. 5.4 Clinical photograph showing ankylosed mandibular right second primary molar

describe this condition to include arrested eruption, buried tooth, impaction, infra-occlusion, incomplete eruption, intrusion, secondary retention, shortened tooth, submerged tooth and suppressed eruption [7]. In children between the ages of 6 and 11, the frequency of ankylosed teeth ranges from eight to 14% with the primary mandibular molars being affected more than the primary maxillary molars [8]. It has been suggested that the mandibular first primary molar is more commonly affected, but since this tooth shows primarily mild infra-occlusion and typically exfoliates on schedule, clinicians may miss this tooth as being ankylosed and therefore believe the mandibular second primary molar to be more commonly affected since it is often more severely infra-occluded [8, 9]. Ankylosed mandibular second primary molars are more likely to be affected bilaterally with the onset occurring later than that of the mandibular first primary molars and with time, the mandibular second molars tend to become more severely infra-occluded than the mandibular first molars [9]. There is an association between ankylosed retained second primary molars and missing permanent successors. In this situation, it has been found that the mandibular second primary molar showed infra-occlusion at 31% as compared to the maxillary second primary molars at 0%. Root resorption occurs in these teeth slowly over time with a decrease in resorption occurring less as the patient age increased [10].

Clinically, ankylosed primary molars will appear lower than the occlusal plane and when percussed they may elicit a dull "cracked teacup" sound [10]. Additionally, depending on the severity of the infra-occlusion, the adjacent teeth may tip into the space created by the seemingly sinking ankylosed tooth and the opposing tooth may supra-erupt into the space [11]. Radiographically, a step in the occlusal plane is observed with the possibility of an angular defect of the alveolar bone angled towards the ankylosed tooth (Fig. 5.5) [8, 10].

Based on the amount of infra-occlusion, ankylosis/submergence has been classified as slight, moderate and severe. Teeth diagnosed as having slight ankylosis, the amount of infra-occlusion measures less than 2 mm, those diagnosed with moderate present with the infra-occlusion at the interproximal contact area and those with severe, the infra-occlusion is well below the interproximal contact area [10].

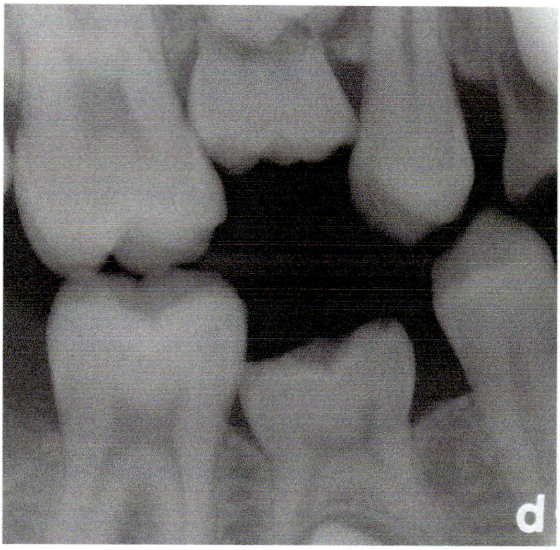

Fig. 5.5 Bitewing radiograph revealing ankylosis of maxillary and mandibular second primary molars

5.3.2 Etiology

The cause of ankylosis is unknown, but multiple theories exist and include a genetic or congenital gap in the periodontal membrane, excessive masticatory pressure or trauma, or a disturbance of local metabolism [7]. Trauma and genetics may be the most significant considerations since with traumatically avulsed anterior permanent teeth; the replanted tooth will usually become ankylosed due to the trauma placed on the periodontal ligament [10]. Even though this explanation seems plausible, it does not explain the tendency for ankyloses to occur in mandibular primary molar teeth. Therefore, one can look to a genetic cause since there is a higher frequency of infra-occluded/ankylosed teeth in siblings [10].

5.3.3 Treatment/Management

Ankylosed primary molars affect occlusal development by complicating the eruption and development of the permanent dentition [12]. There are many treatment options to include extraction and space maintenance, extraction and orthodontic space closure, restorative treatment to build the submerged tooth to the proper height and form, and observation only. Careful assessment of patients with retained primary teeth should occur and all available treatment options considered [13].

Treatment options include:

- Observation is the treatment of choice for at least 6 months according to a systematic review performed by Tieu et al. [8]. In this review, they explored the question of when to extract and when to monitor. The authors of this study discovered that most ankylosed primary molars present with mild to moderate infraocclusion that progresses over time and found that the evidence suggests the appropriate clinical action for these teeth is to monitor for 6 to 12 months after the expected time of exfoliation [8].

- Restoration of the infra-occluded tooth with a good root (not resorbed) and crown (not compromised by caries or defective) is accomplished with composite resin or stainless-steel crowns. Restoring these teeth helps prevent tipping of adjacent teeth and supra eruption of opposing teeth [13].
- If the succedaneous tooth is present, extraction and placement of a space maintainer can be useful to allow the permanent tooth to erupt without the chance of the adjacent teeth erupting into the space (Fig. 5.6).
  - Lower lingual holding arch (LLHA) is used in the situation where both mandibular primary second molars are infra-occluded to the point where mesial tipping of the mandibular permanent molars is occurring. In this situation, both of the mandibular primary second molars are extracted, and then bands are fitted to the mandibular first permanent molars for fabrication of a LLHA. Once cemented onto the molars, the lingual arch wire by contacting the permanent mandibular incisors will prevent mesial tipping of the mandibular first permanent molars allowing the eruption of the succedaneous teeth (second premolars) [9]. Care must be taken to place this appliance after the eruption of the mandibular permanent incisors, to ensure that the lingual archwire does not interfere with the eruption of these teeth (Fig. 5.7).

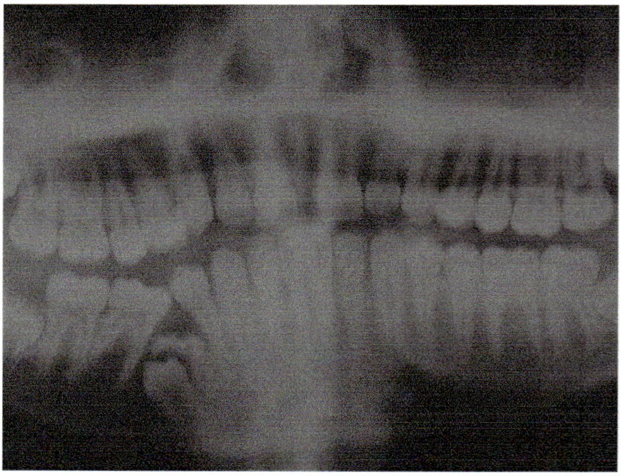

Fig. 5.6 Panoramic radiograph revealing the consequence of a unsupervised ankylosed mandibular right second primary molar

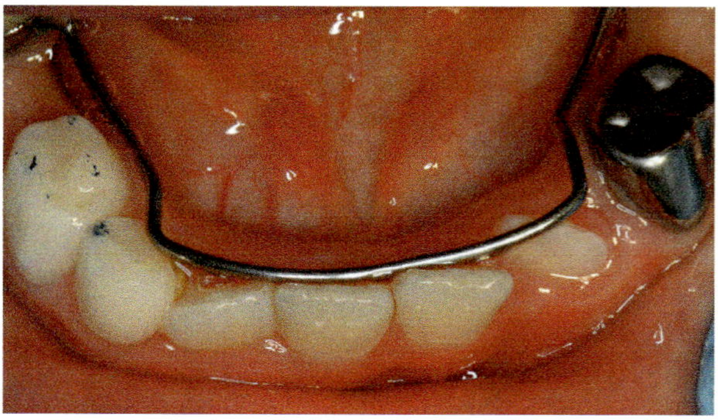

Fig. 5.7 Clinical photograph showing lower lingual holding arch impeding eruption of mandibular left permanent lateral incisor

 - Distal shoe space maintainer is used in situations where the mandibular second primary molar is severely infra-occluded with the mandibular first permanent molar actively erupting. Since the mandibular first permanent molar erupts in a mesial-lingual direction, the infra-occluded mandibular primary second molar cannot adequately guide it into it's normal occlusal position. Therefore, the recommended treatment in this situation is to extract the infra-occluded mandibular second primary molar and fit a band to the mandibular first primary molar with an extension arm engaging the mesial of the erupting first permanent molar that acts as an adequate guide for its eruption [12].
- Extraction and space maintainer if the succedaneous tooth is not present and implant planned. However, the provider should take care with this treatment option since it has been found that the alveolar ridge narrows by 25% in the 4 years following extraction of retained lower primary second molars leading to compromised future restorative management with dental implants [13].
- Extraction and orthodontic space closure if the succedaneous tooth is not present. This is most favorable when crowding exists and an extraction is necessary in order to align the arch orthodontically [13].

5.4 Ectopic Eruption of Maxillary First Permanent Molars

5.4.1 Description

Ectopic eruption of the maxillary first permanent molar is a localized eruption disturbance. The molar erupts with a mesioangular path, becoming entrapped in the distal prominence of the maxillary second primary molar's crown, resulting in atypical resorption of distobuccal root of the maxillary second primary molar (Fig. 5.8) [14].

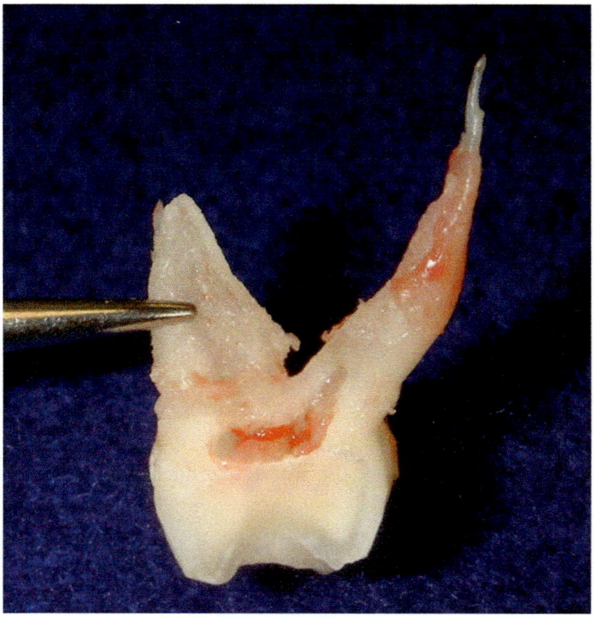

Fig. 5.8 Clinical photograph showing extracted maxillary second primary molar with atypical resorption of the distobuccal root

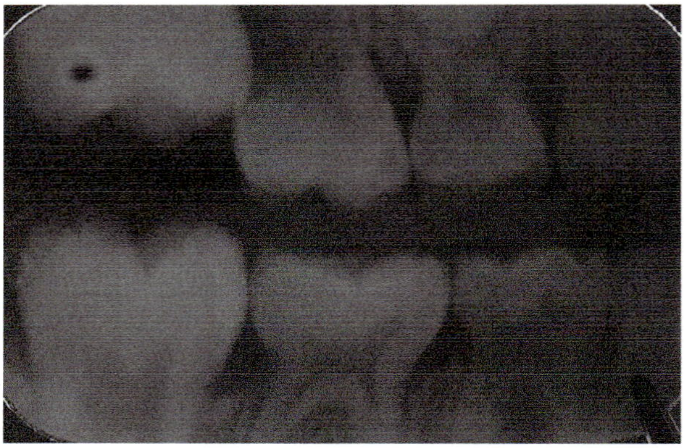

Fig. 5.9 Bitewing radiograph revealing ectopic eruption of erupting maxillary right first permanent molar impacted in distal prominence of the maxillary second primary molar with pulpal exposure

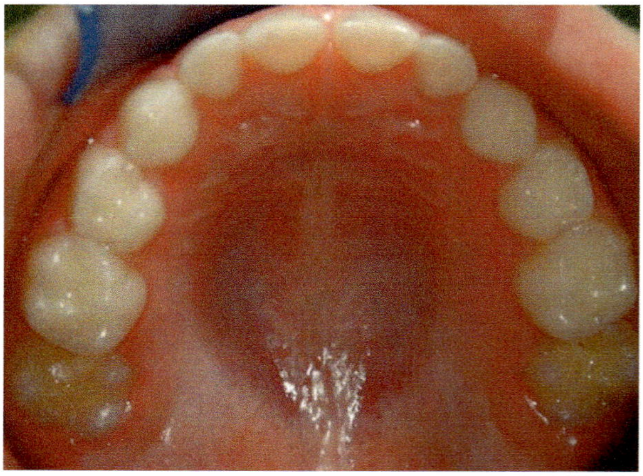

Fig. 5.10 Clinical photograph showing mesial cant of maxillary right and left second primary molars caused by ectopic eruption of the maxillary right and left first permanent molars

This is usually first noted on a routine radiograph prior to eruption of the first permanent molar between five and 7 years of age. In about 14% of cases, pulpal exposure of the second primary molar occurs (Fig. 5.9) [15]. Other than on radiographic exam, the first sign of ectopic eruption of a maxillary first permanent molar may be mesial canting of the maxillary second primary molar (Fig. 5.10). Spontaneous correction with deimpaction and uprighting occurs in 69.4% of cases (Fig. 5.11).

5.4.2 Etiology

The etiology is multifactorial, with causes not well known. Prior to eruption, the tooth germ of the maxillary first permanent molar is oriented downward, backward and outward. A more vertical orientation is assumed during eruption. Without this change in orientation, the impaction under the distobuccal of the adjacent second primary molar results. Larger than average size first permanent molars and a shorter maxilla, with inadequate arch length, have been suggested to contribute to this

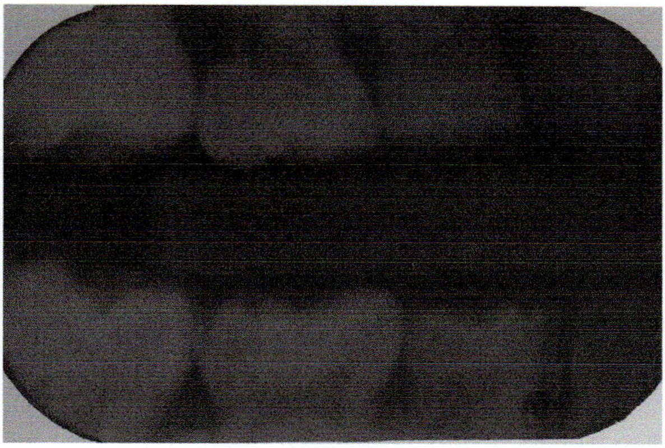

Fig. 5.11 Bitewing radiograph revealing spontaneous correction of ectopic eruption of maxillary right first permanent molar

disturbance. Studies report prevalence to be from 3 to 4.3% of patients, and more common in children with cleft palate. A prevalence of 19.9% has been reported in siblings, suggesting a genetic component. No significant difference between males and females has been reported [15].

5.4.3 Treatment/Management

Intervention is aimed at avoiding premature loss of the second primary molar and continued space loss. If dental and chronologic age correspond, self-correction should occur between 6 and 7 years of age. If self-correction does not occur, treatment is necessary. The goal of intervention is to upright the first permanent molar permitting normal eruption [16]. There are various methods to achieve deimpaction.

- Place a commercial separating spring between the second primary molar and the first permanent molar to de-impact. (Figs. 5.12, 5.13, and 5.14) [16].
- Place a brass ligature wire between the second primary molar and the first permanent molar (Fig. 5.15). The wire is twisted together with a Howe plier, recording the direction of the twist, and the wire is tucked into the embrasure (Figs. 5.16, 5.17). The wire is tightened every 2–3 weeks until it is easily removed after deimpaction has occurred. A periapical radiograph is obtained to evaluate the stability of the second primary molar and its ability to act as a space maintainer [16, 17].
- Separation with an orthodontic elastic separator is typically better tolerated than a separating spring or brass wire. Place an orthodontic elastic separator with waxed dental floss between the second primary molar and first permanent molar to de-impact the first permanent molar (Figs. 5.18, 5.19, 5.20, and 5.21) [16, 18]. The elastic separator will be lost spontaneously with correction or should be removed if still in place after deimpaction has occurred (Fig. 5.22).

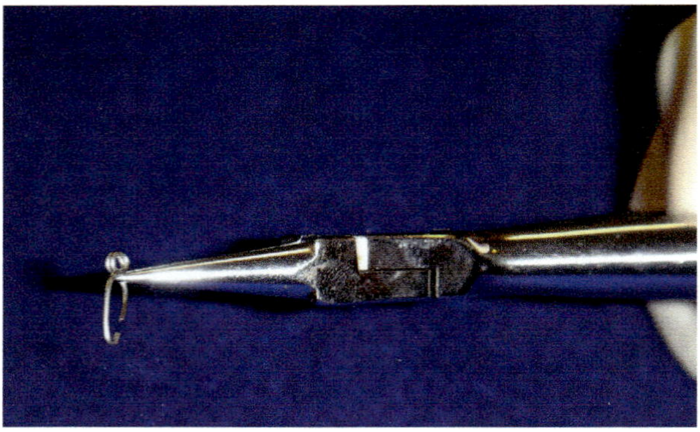

Fig. 5.12 Clinical photograph showing a separating spring

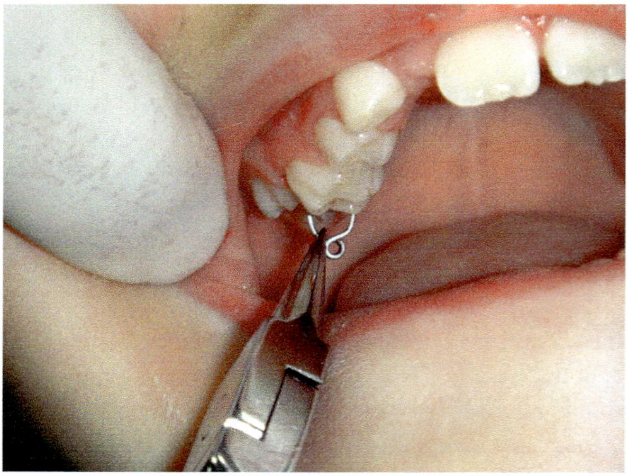

Fig. 5.13 Clinical photograph showing a separating spring being placed to deimpact maxillary first permanent molar

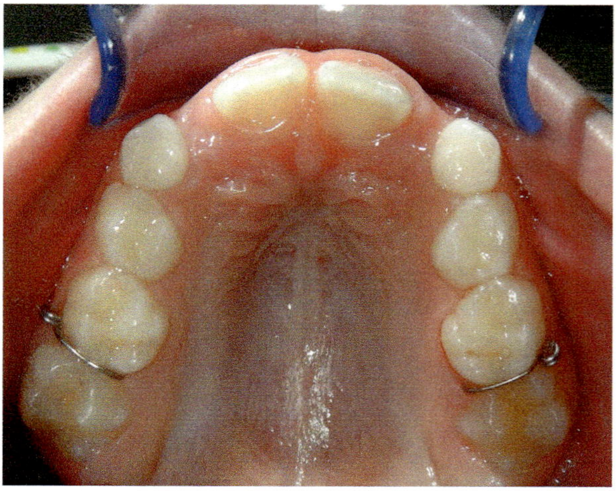

Fig. 5.14 Clinical photograph showing deimpacted maxillary right and left first permanent molars with separating springs

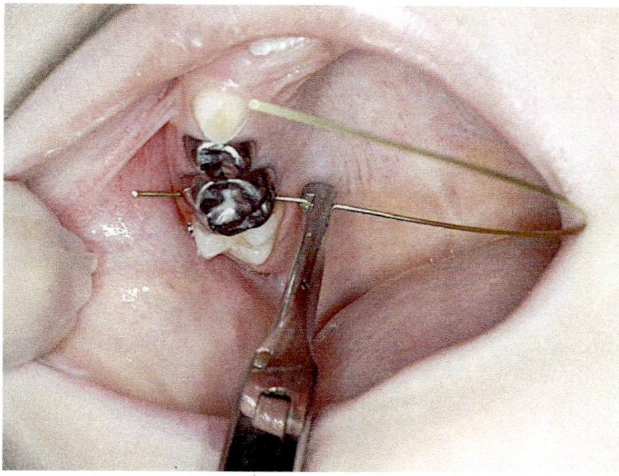

Fig. 5.15 Clinical photograph showing brass wire being placed between impacted maxillary right first permanent molar and maxillary second primary molar from palatal direction

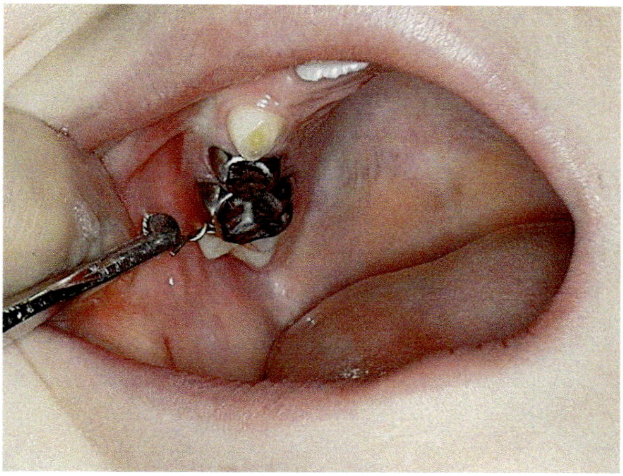

Fig. 5.16 Clinical photograph showing cut brass wire twisted together

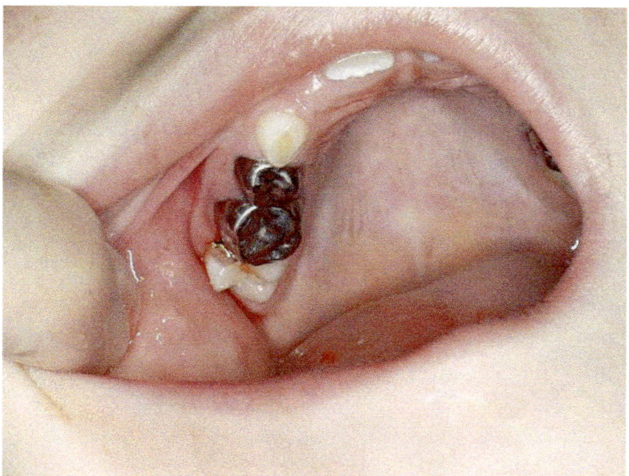

Fig. 5.17 Clinical photograph showing brass wire tucked into the embrasure

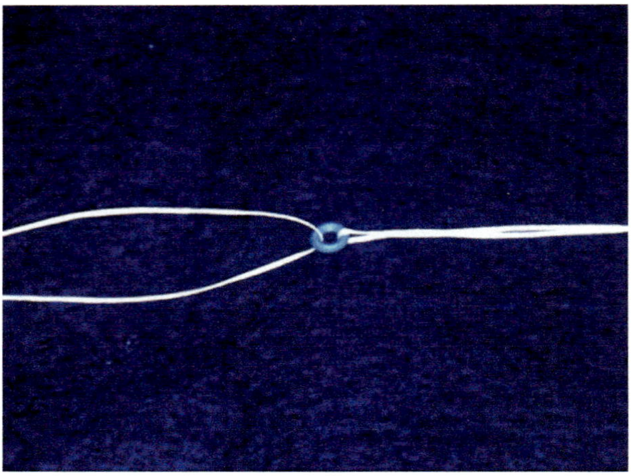

Fig. 5.18 Clinical photograph showing floss in orthodontic elastic separator

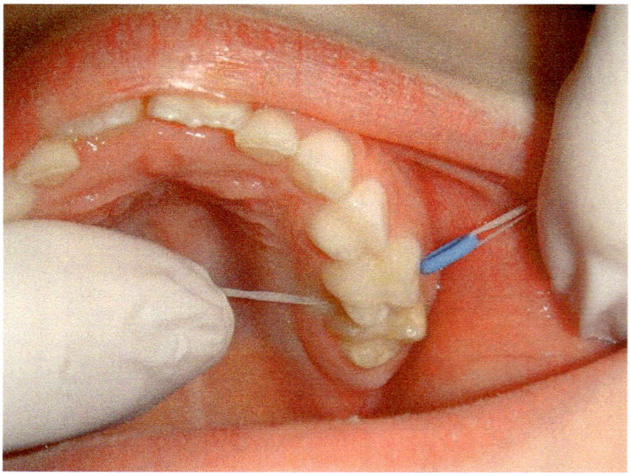

Fig. 5.19 Clinical photograph showing flossing orthodontic elastic separator between impacted maxillary first permanent molar and second primary molar

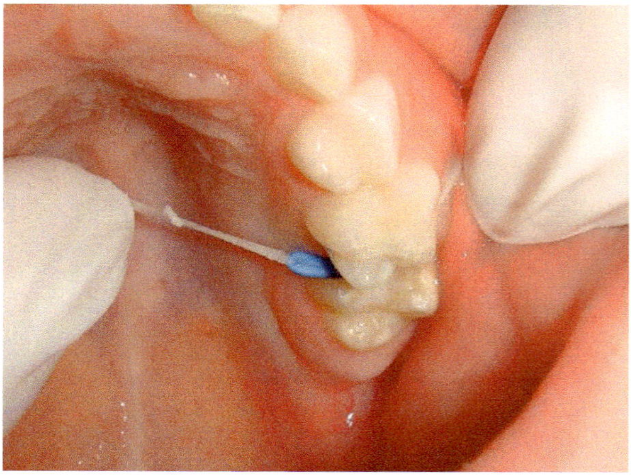

Fig. 5.20 Clinical photograph showing floss and orthodontic elastic separator through contact

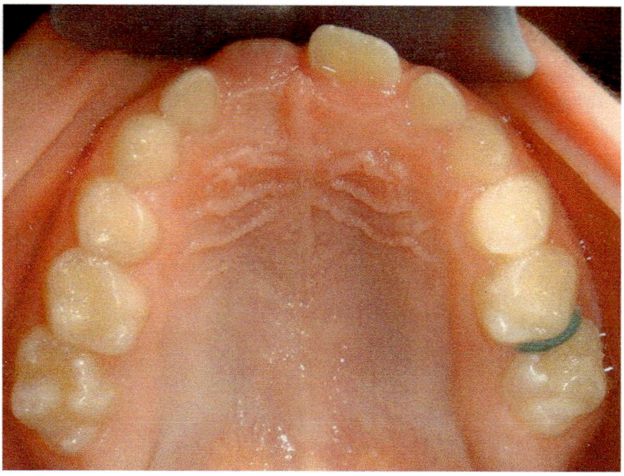

Fig. 5.21 Clinical photograph showing floss removed and orthodontic elastic separator in place

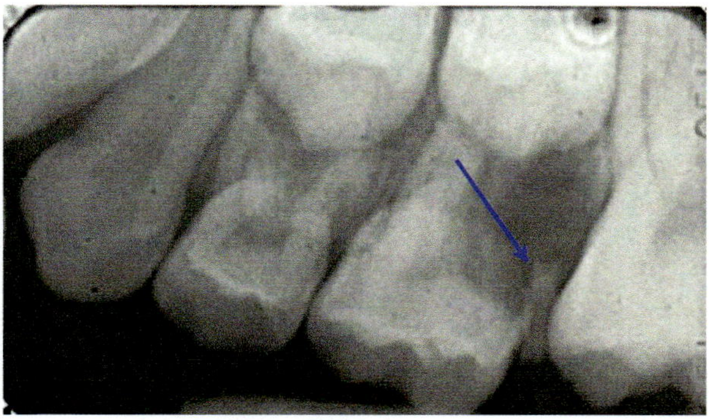

Fig. 5.22 Periapical radiograph revealing deimpacted maxillary first permanent molar with radiopaque orthodontic elastic separator still in place

- Interproximal enamel reduction of the distal of the second primary molar with a 169 L carbide bur in high speed. A wedge between the maxillary second primary molar and the impacted maxillary first permanent molar will protect the mesial of the first permanent molar from inadvertently disking the mesial of the maxillary first permanent molar (Fig. 5.23) [16, 18].
- Active appliance therapy with a Halterman appliance or ectopic spring loaded distalizer if deimpaction cannot be achieved with other methods.
- The Halterman appliance is designed with a mushroom-shaped stainless steel button bonded to the occlusal surface of the impacted first permanent molar. A band with a soldered hook that extends distally is cemented on the second primary molar. A chain elastic is placed between the hook and the button to apply a distal force to the first permanent molar (Fig. 5.24). The ectopic spring loaded distalizer functions similarly to the Halterman appliance, but without the bonded button, which may cause concern regarding swallowing or aspiration. An arm extends distally from a band on the second primary molar to the occlusal surface of the first permanent molar. The arm is bonded to the first permanent molar's

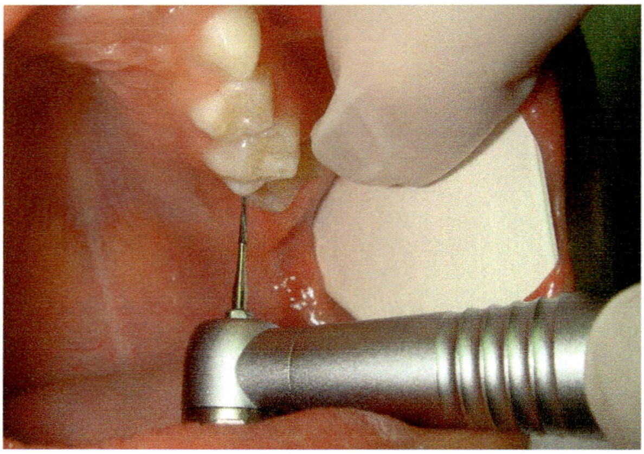

Fig. 5.23 Clinical photograph showing disking the distal surface of maxillary second primary molar to assist spontaneous deimpaction of the maxillary permanent first molar

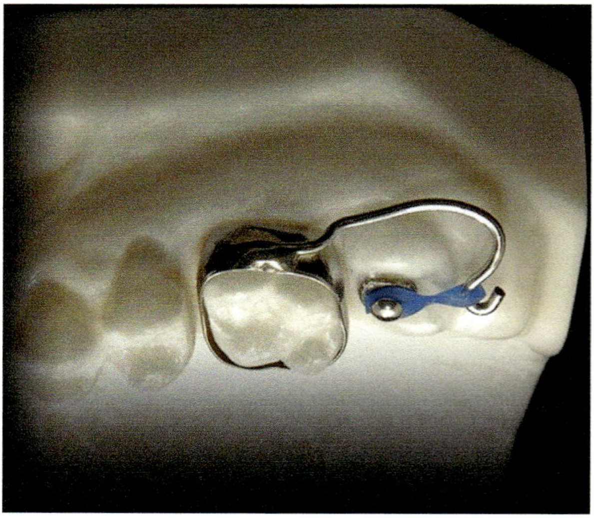

Fig. 5.24 Halterman appliance (Courtesy of QC Orthodontics Lab)

buccal cusp. The appliance is delivered with a coil spring that is compressed and pre-activated. An elastic chain holds the coil passive until the appliance is cemented. Activation occurs when the chain elastic is cut and removed (Fig. 5.25).

The second primary molar is maintained as long as possible to hold the space for the maxillary second premolar. When the second primary molar becomes symptomatic, mobile, abscessed or advanced root resorption has occurred, extraction is necessary (Fig. 5.26).

A reverse band and loop is usually the first space maintainer that can be used; since the first permanent molar is not adequately erupted to band. The first primary molar is banded with a loop that extends distally to the partially erupted first permanent molar (Fig. 5.27). Once the first permanent molar has adequately erupted to fit and cement an orthodontic band, a transpalatal or Nance space maintainer can be fabricated for space control (Figs. 5.28 and 5.29). If extraction must be performed

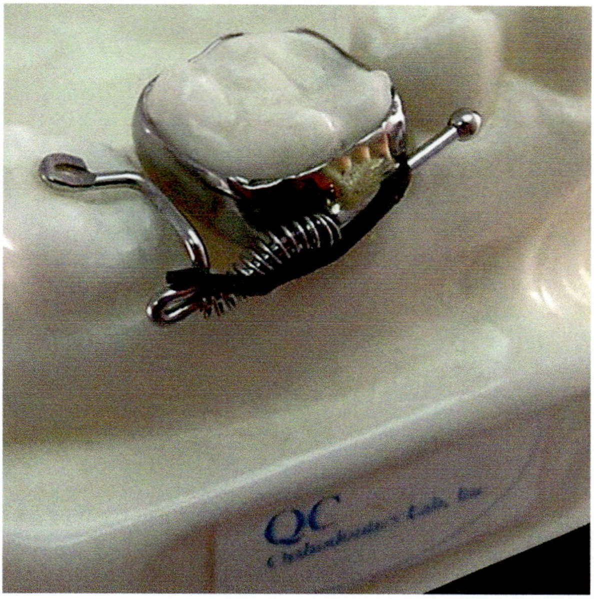

Fig. 5.25 Ectopic spring loaded distalizer appliance (Courtesy of QC Orthodontics Lab)

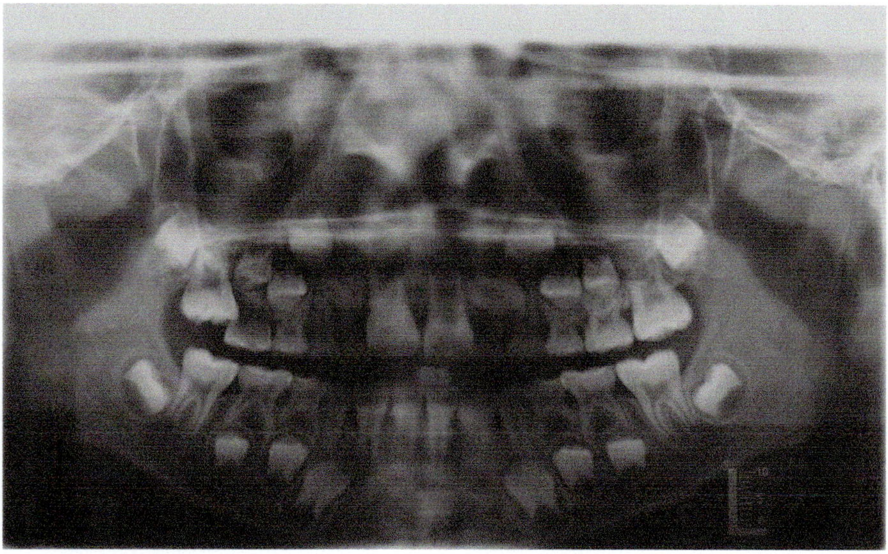

Fig. 5.26 Panoramic radiograph revealing advanced root resorption of maxillary right second primary molar secondary to ectopic eruption of maxillary right first permanent molar

prior to the eruption of the permanent molar, a distal shoe space maintainer is the appliance of choice (Fig. 5.30). The caregiver is advised that if space loss occurred prior to the ability to intervene, that orthodontic treatment may be necessary to regain the lost space.

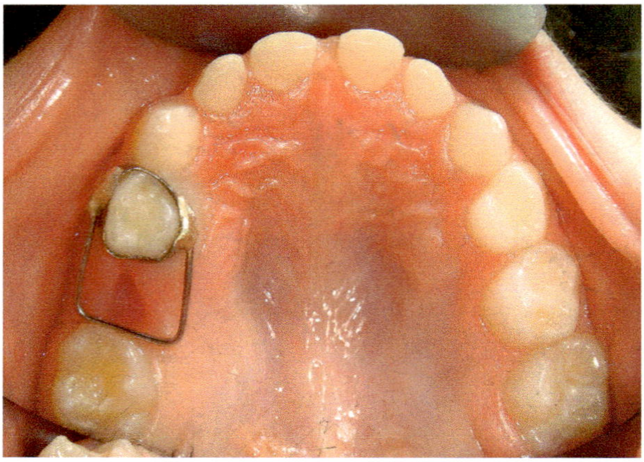

Fig. 5.27 Clinical photograph showing band and loop space maintainer to maintain space for maxillary second premolar

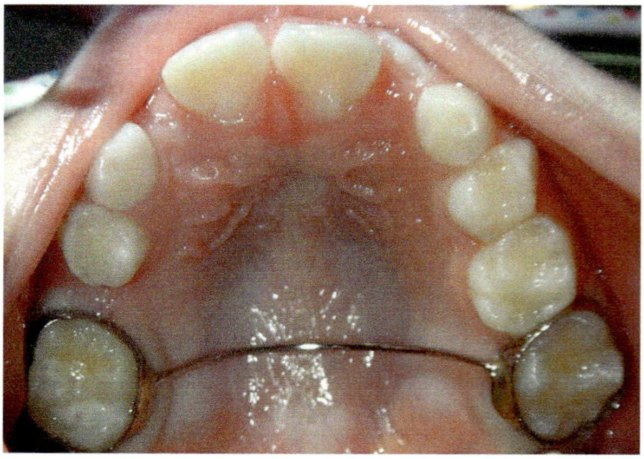

Fig. 5.28 Clinical photograph showing transpalatal appliance for premature unilateral loss of maxillary second primary molar

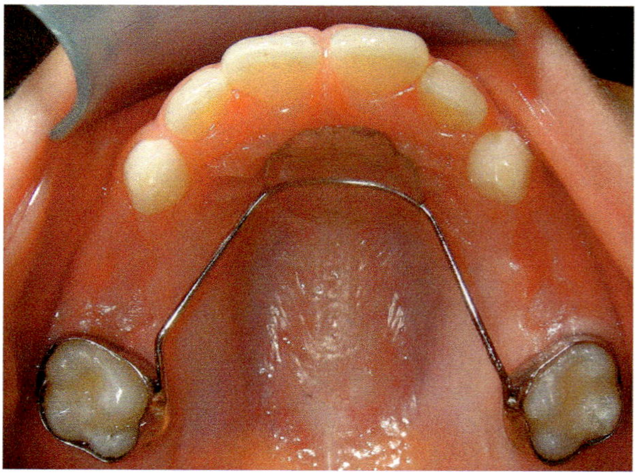

Fig. 5.29 Clinical photograph showing Nance appliance for premature bilateral loss of maxillary second primary molars

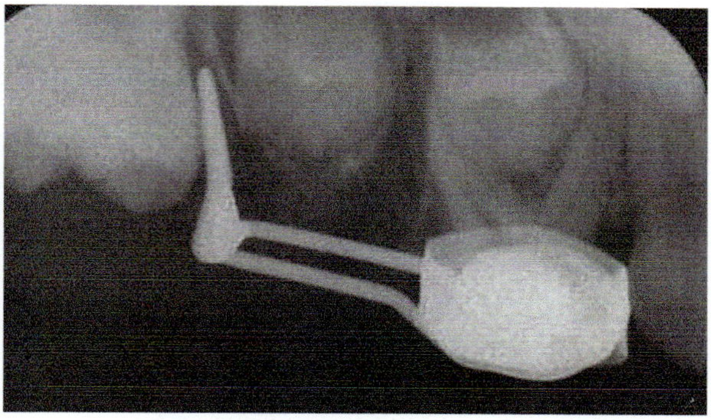

Fig. 5.30 Periapical radiograph of distal shoe appliance for premature loss of maxillary second primary molar and unerupted first permanent molar

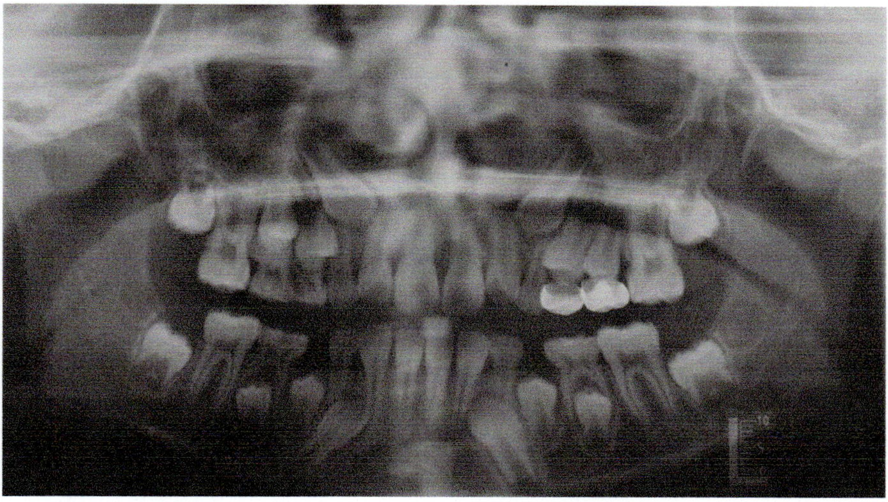

Fig. 5.31 Panoramic radiograph revealing ectopic position of maxillary right and left permanent canines

5.5 Ectopic Eruption and Impaction of Maxillary Permanent Canines

5.5.1 Description

Displacement of maxillary permanent canines may occur in the maxillary arch (Fig. 5.31). The maxillary permanent canines are second to third molars as the most often impacted teeth [19]. Lateral incisors, adjacent to palatally displaced canines, are associated with anomalies such as smaller in length with roots smaller in width, particularly in the buccolingual dimension, peg-shape (Fig. 5.32) (As discussed in Chap. 3), and agenesis. Delayed dental development has also been linked to palatally displaced

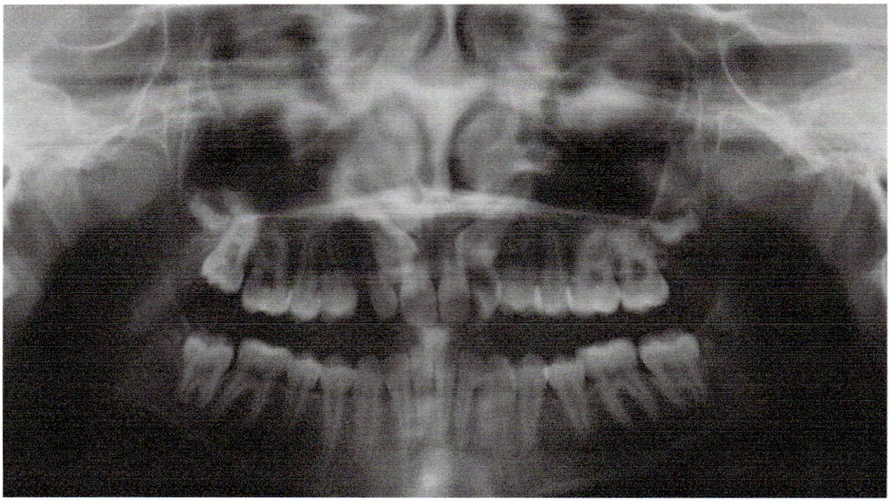

Fig. 5.32 Panoramic radiograph revealing ectopic position of maxillary permanent canines associated with microdontia of maxillary permanent lateral incisors

maxillary permanent canines [20]. Maxillary permanent canines normally erupt at age 11 ± 2 years [18]. With digital palpation of the alveolar process, high in the buccal sulcus, absence of a permanent canine bulge at 9 or 10 years of age may indicate displacement or ectopic position of these teeth [14, 16]. Continued digital monitoring is advisable; since position of unerupted canine(s) may change from upright to ectopic later during development (Figs. 5.33a, b). Displacement is typically to the palatal [21]. Dental age versus chronological age should be considered when evaluating the canine bulge; since the bulge may be absent at age 10 with delayed dental development. Knowledge of sequence of eruption is important to understand the pathway for guidance and proper alignment of the maxillary canine. The maxillary lateral incisor and the maxillary first premolar precede the eruption of the maxillary canine, assisting the path of eruption. If the canine is just buccal to the alignment of the maxillary arch, with adequate space and no impediment, normal eruption should follow [19].

5.5.2 Etiology

The high developmental location and earlier development of the crown have been suggested as reasons for displacement. The eruption path of the permanent canines is a distance of 22 mm from the floor of the orbit to the final position in the dental arch, contributing to an ectopic course [19]. Insufficient arch length with resultant crowding usually causes buccal displacement, however one study showed that in 85% of palatal impaction cases, adequate space was available for eruption. Two theories of guidance and genetics cite causes for this eruption disturbance. Eruption of the maxillary canine typically occurs with the root of the adjacent lateral incisor guiding the tooth into position. With microdontia or agenesis, guidance is absent. The genetic

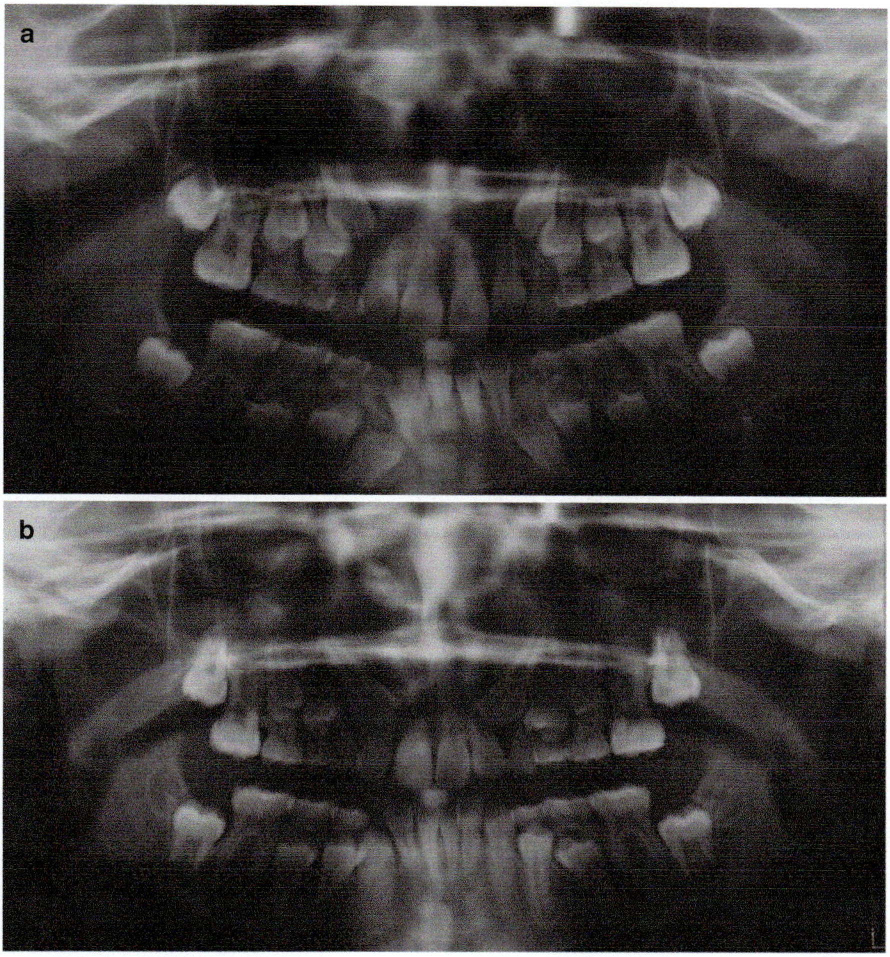

Fig. 5.33 (**a**) Panoramic radiograph revealing suitable position of maxillary right and left permanent canines at age 8 years 9 months. (**b**) Panoramic radiograph of same patient revealing significant change in position of maxillary right and left permanent canines at age 11 years 8 months

theory suggests genetically linked abnormalities such as tooth shape, number, structure and size as contributory [21]. Becker and Chaushu concur, adding two additional causes for impaction of maxillary permanent canines and classifying the causes into four distinct groupings: disturbance of normal development of the incisors, hereditary or genetic factors, local pathology, and local hard tissue obstruction [19].

- Disturbance of normal development of the incisors is understood with a review of the normal eruption and alignment of the maxillary incisors, first described by Broadbent more than 70 years ago. With adequate space, the permanent central incisors erupt with a wide diastema. The permanent laterals move incisally down the distal aspect of the central incisors, closing the intra-coronal space between the centrals. The permanent canines are guided into position as they erupt along the distal aspect of the roots of the permanent lateral incisors. Upon complete eruption of the permanent canines, if adequate space is present in the anterior segment of the maxillary arch, the mid-line diastema is closed and the crowns of the six permanent incisors contact interproximally. With a small, pegged or missing lateral incisor, the incidence of palatal displacement is increased due to absence of guidance for a normal eruption path. An anomalous lateral incisor was associated with canine impaction 7 times more frequently than on the contralateral side with congenital absence.

- Genetic and hereditary factors are accompanied with inconsistencies. For genetics to be solely responsible for impaction of maxillary permanent canines, one would expect bilateral involvement in the majority of cases. However, literature review indicates 60–75% to be unilateral. In comparing monozygous (identical) and dizygous (fraternal) twins, similar degrees of canine impaction were found in both groups, reinforcing a non-genetic etiology. An anomalous permanent lateral incisor has been shown to be associated 7 times more often with an impacted canine than a congenitally missing permanent lateral incisor. Congenital absence of a permanent lateral incisor is a stronger genetic trait than anomalous incisors. Anomalous incisors, more often accompanying impacted canines, represent more of partial expression or incomplete penetrance, also supporting a non-genetic etiology [19].
- Local pathology, in the form of a granuloma, may occur with carious non-vital primary canines, severe attrition or post-traumatic injury. This soft tissue inflammatory lesion can deflect the eruption path of the permanent canine or cease the eruption. A dentigerous cyst can also cause deflection from the normal path of eruption (Fig. 5.34).

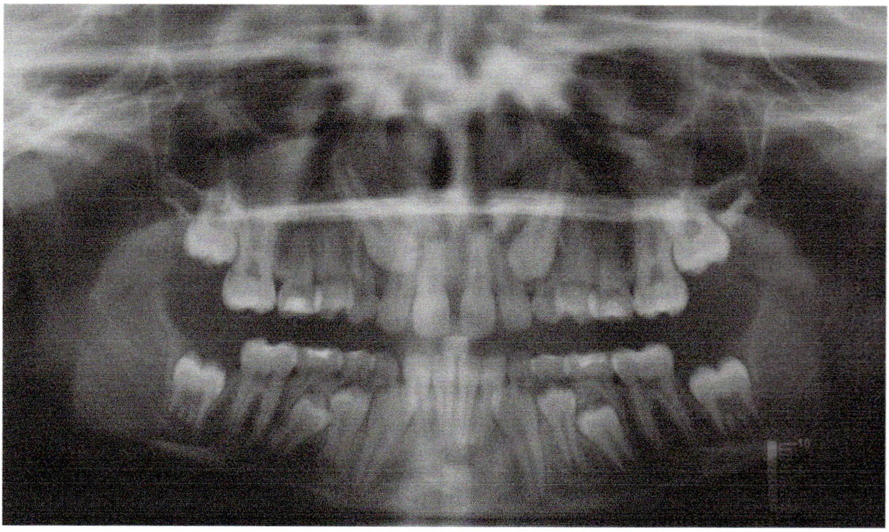

Fig. 5.34 Panoramic radiograph revealing a dentigerous cyst causing ectopic eruption of maxillary left permanent canine and palatal position of the ectopic maxillary right permanent canine

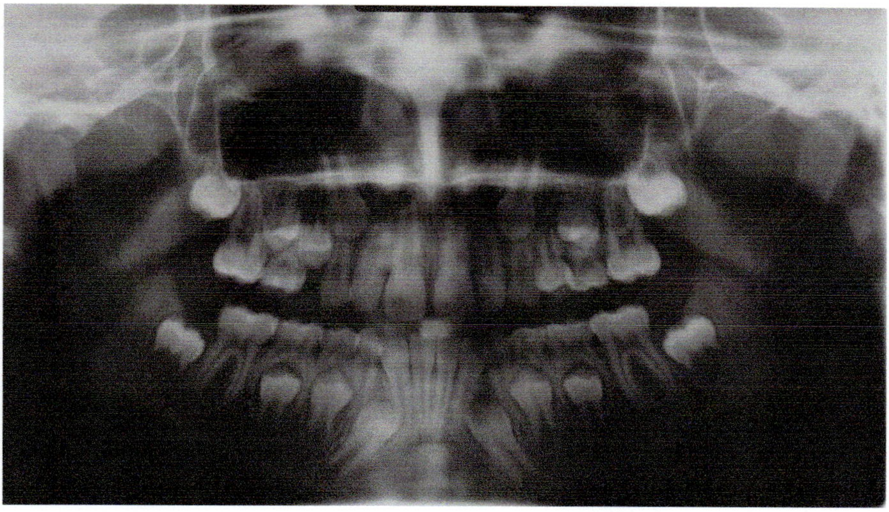

Fig. 5.35 Panoramic radiograph revealing unresorbed roots on maxillary right and left primary canines associated with palatal displacement of maxillary right and left permanent canines

- Local hard tissue obstruction may be due to an odontoma, a supernumerary, a palatal root of a first premolar that erupted with a mesiobuccal rotation, or a long, unresorbed root of a primary canine (Fig. 5.35).

The guidance theory and the genetic theory concur that some genetically directed factors such as anomalous of missing lateral incisors, dental delay, and spaced dentitions contribute to palatal displacement of maxillary canines by loss of eruptive guidance, strongly suggesting that the eruption path of the maxillary permanent canines does not appear to be directed by genetics but rather by guidance [19].

One circumstance strongly suggests heredity. The teeth are arranged in the embryonic dental lamina in a specific order. The apex of the canine's root shows the original location of the tooth germ. Apical mislocation is genetically directed and consequently seen bilaterally; since the right and left sides of one's body should be identical. Although variations due to genetic expression may occur, reflected in the orientation of the long axes of the canines, the location of the apex is likely to be bilaterally comparable. The roots of these canines are displaced distally and palatal to the premolars. Because this circumstance does not result from impeded guidance, interceptive treatment with extraction or orthodontic intervention to open space in the arch cannot provide resolution. Surgical exposure with orthodontic force will be required to bring these canines into the arch. Cone-beam computerized tomography is preferable to conventional radiography for diagnosis of the location of the apices.

Distal displacement of mandibular second premolars is an anomaly shown to be associated with palatally displaced canines (Fig. 5.36) [22]. Early identification of distally displaced mandibular second premolar(s) on radiographic examination can alert the clinician to the possibility of palatally displaced canines.

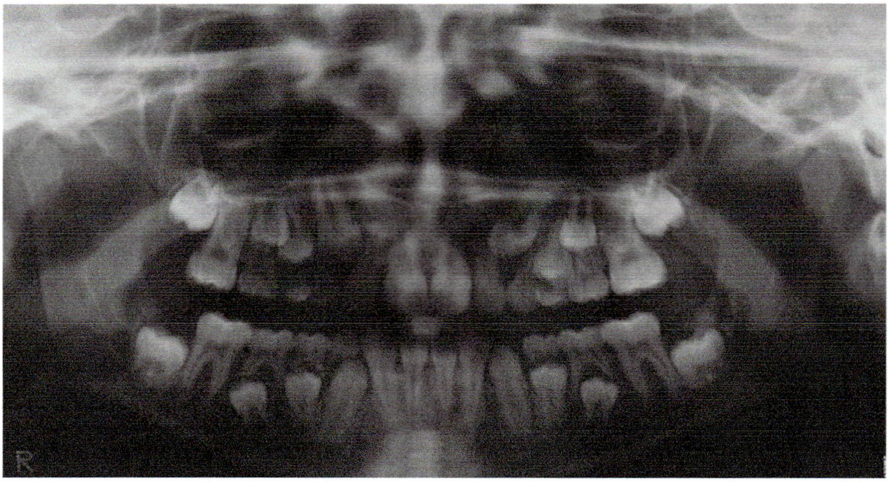

Fig. 5.36 Panoramic radiograph revealing distally displaced mandibular right and left second premolars and ectopic position of maxillary right and left permanent canines

5.5.3 Treatment/Management

Adolescence is considered to be the optimal time for treatment [11]. Treatment is aimed to not only change the path of eruption of the maxillary permanent canine, but to avoid root resorption of the adjacent lateral incisor (Figs. 5.37 and 5.38) [16, 23]. Panoramic or periapical radiographic examination confirms the position of the permanent canine. Two periapical radiographs, taken from two different views, is a common method (Clark's rule) to diagnose palatally displaced canines. Cone beam computed tomography is deemed to be more diagnostic for determining the location of the canines and identification of root resorption on the adjacent lateral incisors [24].

In the majority of patients, spontaneous change in the eruption path of the maxillary permanent canine can occur with a change in the environmental conditions.

Adjunctive use of cervical headgear in order to maintain space in the maxillary arch significantly improved intraosseous canine position [23]. Increasing arch space in the area with orthodontic treatment or rapid palatal expansion, or extraction of first premolars are treatment modalities to alleviate anterior crowding that may improve eruption path [19]. Extraction of primary canines is often cited as successful intervention with better positional changes and more decreased eruption time (Figs. 5.39 and 5.40) [19, 23, 25]. If one-half root formation is radiographically evident on the maxillary first premolar (Fig. 5.41), adding extraction of the first primary molar may stimulate eruption of the first premolar, providing a guide for the eruption path of the permanent canine (Fig. 5.42) [23]. For palatally displaced canines, timely, interceptive extraction of the maxillary primary canines aides spontaneous eruption [16, 25]. Extraction of the primary canine has also been shown to be an effective method to aid eruption of the permanent canine if the primary canine is impeding the eruption of the permanent canine.

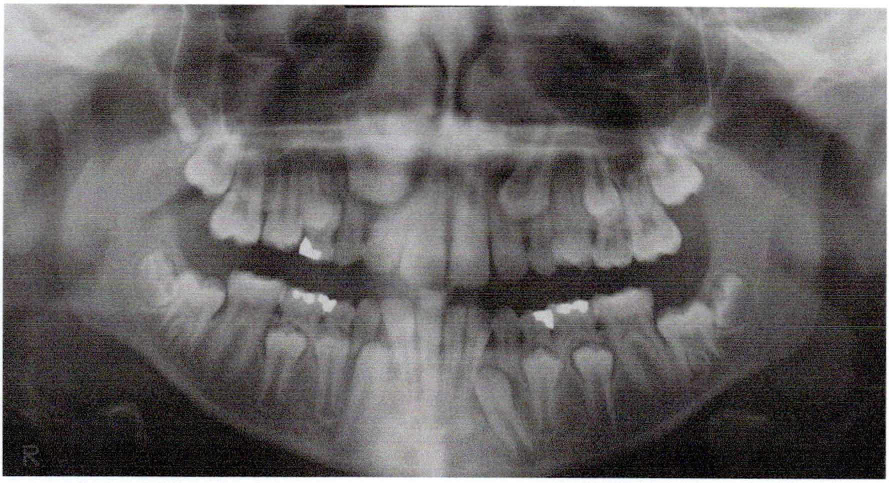

Fig. 5.37 Panoramic radiograph revealing impending root resorption of maxillary right permanent lateral incisor with ectopic eruption of maxillary right permanent canine

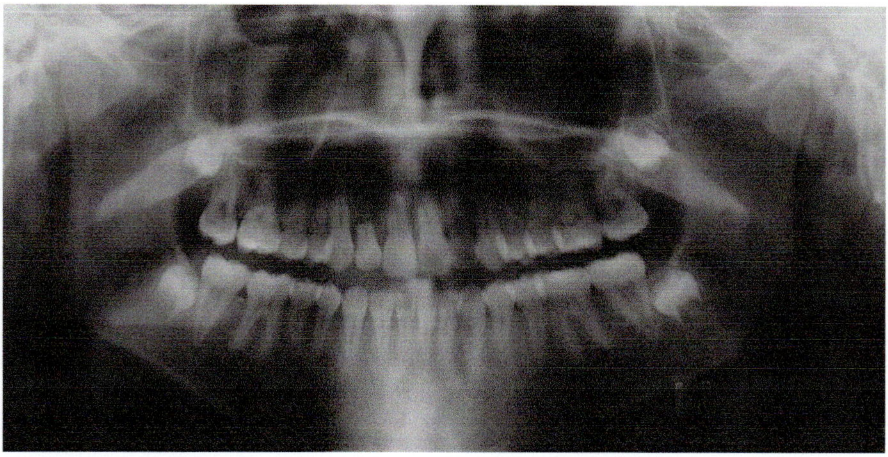

Fig. 5.38 Panoramic radiograph post-orthodontic intervention revealing root resorption of maxillary right permanent lateral incisor caused by ectopic eruption of maxillary right permanent canine prior to orthodontic intervention

Two methods of surgical exposure are used for correction of palatally impacted ectopic maxillary canines: closed exposure and open exposure. With closed exposure, after the first 6–9 months of alignment and creating space, the palatally impacted canine is surgically uncovered and an auxiliary attachment is bonded to the tooth (Fig. 5.43). Orthodontic force with ballista loops or a gold chain is then used for traction to drag the impacted maxillary permanent canine(s) into the edentulous site (Figs. 5.44 and 5.45) [11, 26]. Alternatively, with open exposure, the impacted

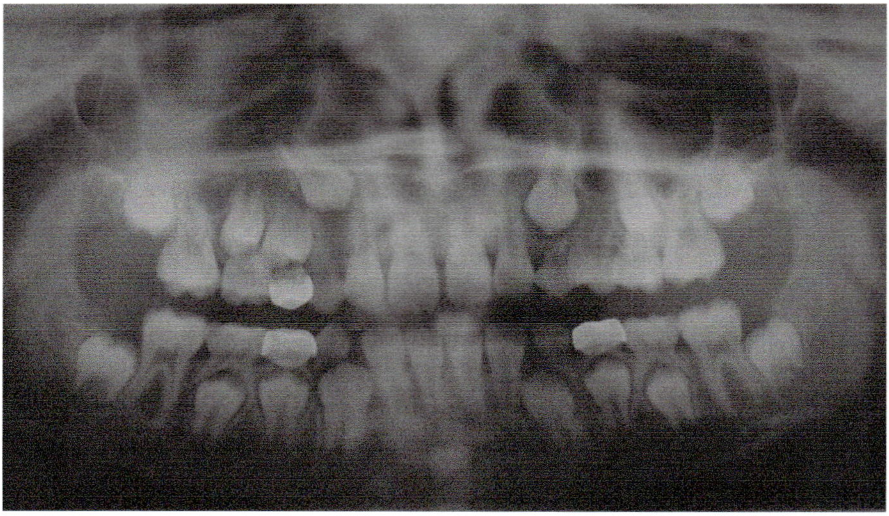

Fig. 5.39 Panoramic radiograph revealing ectopic orientation of maxillary right permanent canine

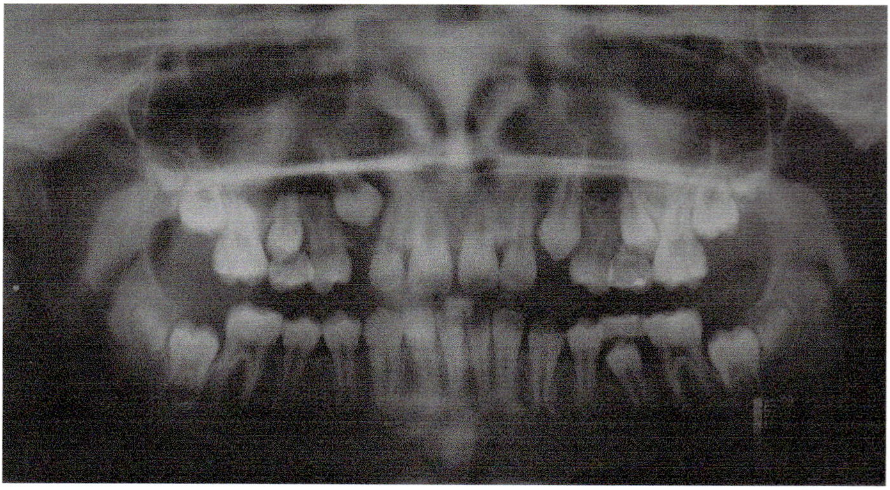

Fig. 5.40 Panoramic radiograph revealing correcting orientation of unerupted maxillary right permanent canine post extraction of maxillary right primary canine

canine(s) may be uncovered prior to beginning orthodontic treatment in the late mixed dentition. A full thickness mucoperiosteal flap is performed, exposing the impacted canine. All bone surrounding the crown is removed up to the cementoenamel junction to facilitate eruption. The flap is put back in place and a hole is created in the flap. The impacted canine freely erupts in about 6–8 months without orthodontic assistance. Once the tooth has erupted to the level of the occlusal plane,

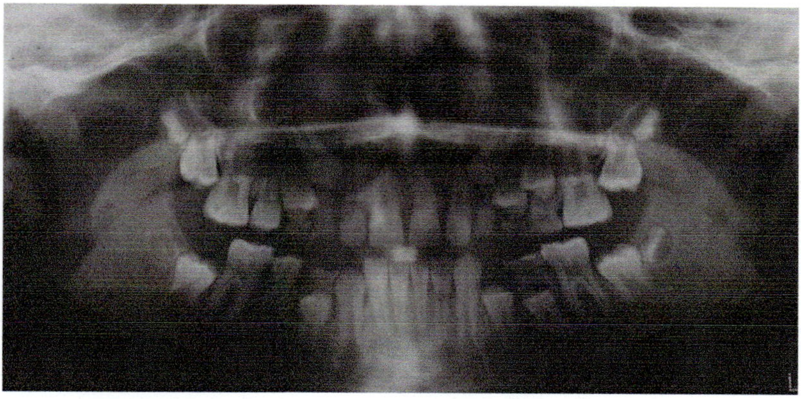

Fig. 5.41 Panoramic radiograph revealing ectopic eruption of maxillary right and left permanent canines and one-half root formation of the maxillary first premolars

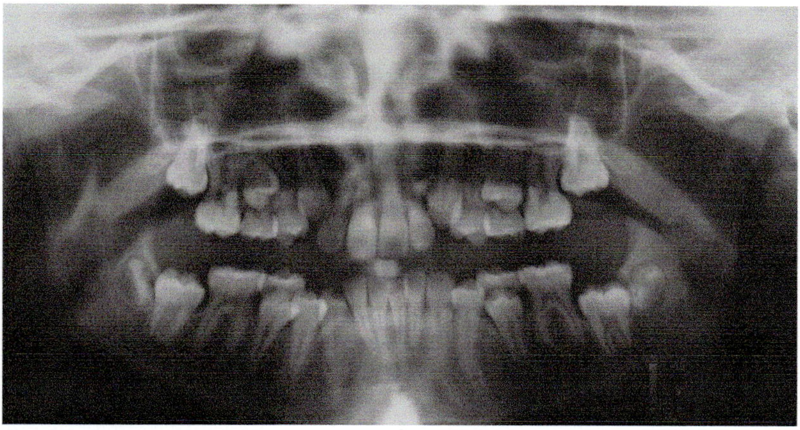

Fig. 5.42 Panoramic radiograph of same patient in Fig. 5.33b revealing corrected orientation of maxillary permanent canines 13 months post extraction of maxillary primary canines and first primary molars

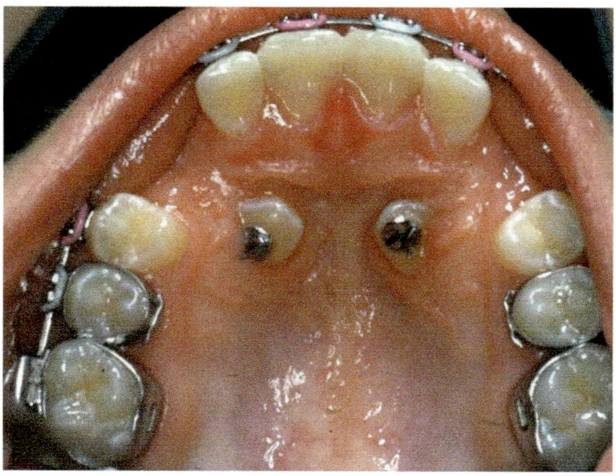

Fig. 5.43 Clinical photograph showing auxiliary attachments on surgically exposed maxillary right and left permanent canines

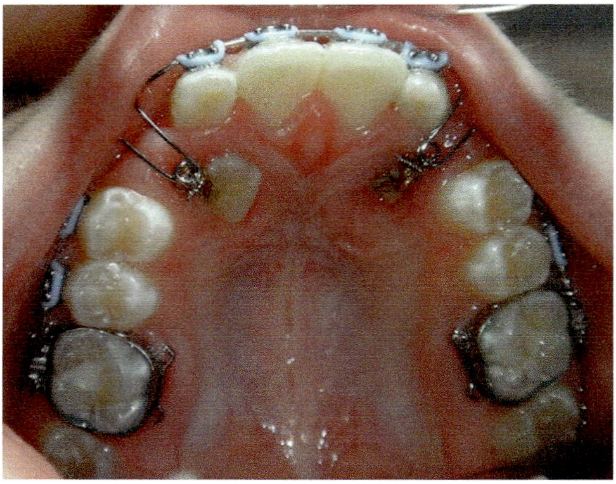

Fig. 5.44 Clinical photograph showing ballista loops on surgically exposed maxillary right and left permanent canines (Courtesy of Dr. John F Buzzatto)

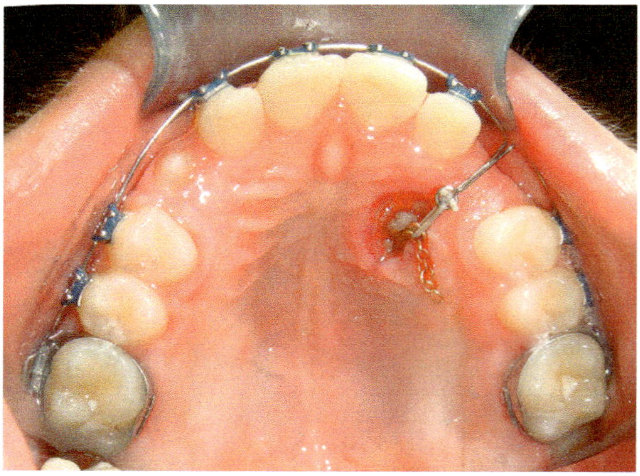

Fig. 5.45 Clinical photograph showing gold chain on surgically exposed maxillary left permanent canine

a bracket is placed for movement through the bone and alignment in the arch [26]. Both approaches require good oral hygiene and compliance wearing fixed orthodontic appliances during prolonged treatment time. In some cases, exposure may not be a viable treatment option if the impacted canine is in a horizontal position above the apices of the adjacent teeth and in close proximity to the midline [11].

5.6 Dental Transposition

5.6.1 Description

This anomaly is an extreme type of ectopic eruption manifested by the interchanged position of two permanent teeth. Typically the maxillary canine and the first

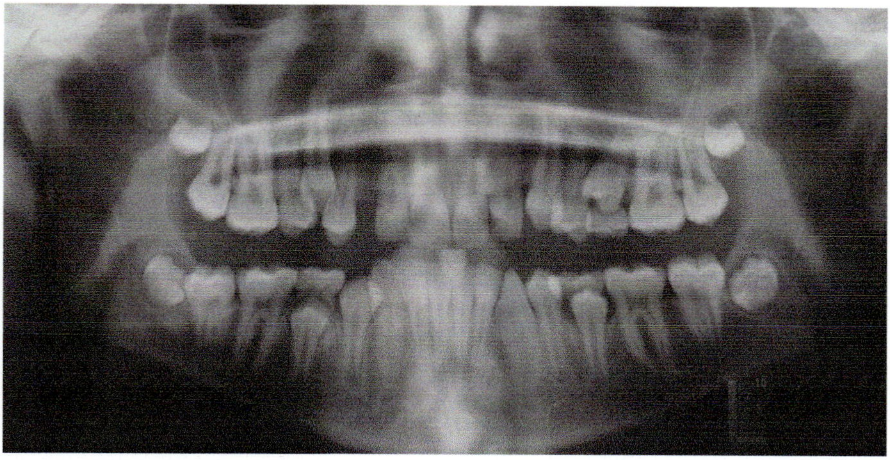

Fig. 5.46 Panoramic radiograph revealing transposition of maxillary right permanent canine and first premolar

premolar have positional interchange (Fig. 5.46). As commonly occurs, additional anomalies are associated with transposition. Permanent lateral incisors smaller than the norm or missing, over-retained primary canines, impaction of central incisors and permanent canines, missing maxillary and mandibular second premolars, and significant rotation of adjacent teeth are accompanying presentations, typically occurring on the same side as the transposition. Similarities between the dental anomalies in persons with clefts of the lip and palate and transposition have brought speculation that similar genetic or local factors could be responsible for the concomitant anomalies. Transposition is more common in females, usually unilateral, and on the left side of the arch [27, 28].

5.6.2 Etiology

This anomaly may involve interchange of the involved teeth in the dental lamina, multifactorial genetic factors, or a traumatic injury involving a primary tooth resulting in of the permanent incisor root.

5.6.3 Treatment/Management

The transposed teeth may be orthodontically moved to the proper position in the arch, reshaped after eruption or extracted with orthodontically assisted space closure [27].

References

1. Wang CH, Lin YT, Lin YT (2017) A survey of natal and neonatal teeth in newborn infants. J Formos Med Assoc 116:193–196
2. Machado de Almeida C, Gomide MR (1996) Prevalence of natal/neonatal teeth in cleft lip and palate infants. Cleft Palate Craniofac J 33(4):297–299
3. Cunha RF, Carrilho Boer FA, Dias Torriani D, Gabeline Frossard WT (2001) Natal and neonatal teeth: review of the literature. Pediatr Dent 23(2):158–162
4. Waage NS, Baker S, Sedano HO (2009) Pediatric condition associated with compromised airway: part 1 – congenital. Pediatr Dent 31(3):236–248
5. Buchanan S, Jenkins CR (1997) Riga-Fedes syndrome: Natal or neonatal teeth associated with tongue ulceration. Case report. Aust Dent J 42(4):225–228
6. Kim SH, Cho YA, Nam OHN, Kim MS, Choi SC, Lee HS (2016) Complication after extraction of natal teeth with continued growth of a dental papilla. Pediatr Dent 38(7):E137–EE14
7. Kurol J (1981) Infraocclusion of primary molars: an epidemiologic and familial study. Community Dent Oral Epidemiol 9:94–102
8. Tieu LD, Walker SL, Major MP, Flores-Mir C (2013) Management of ankylosed primary molars with premolar successors. JADA 144(6):602–611
9. Messer LB, Cline JT (1980) Ankylosed primary molars: results and treatment recommendations from an eight-year longitudinal study. Pediatr Dent 2(1):37–47
10. Kennedy DB (2009) Review: treatment strategies for ankylosed primary molars. Eur Arch Paediatr Dent 10(4):201–210
11. Husain J, Burden D, McSherry P et al (2012) National clinical guidelines for management of the palatally ectopic maxillary canine. Br Dent J 213(4):171–176
12. Kirshenblatt S, Kulkarni GV (2011) Complications of surgical extraction of ankylosed primary teeth and distal shoe space maintainers. J Dent Child 78(1):57–61
13. Robinson S, Chan MFW-Y (2009) New teeth from old: treatment options for retained primary teeth. Br Dent J 207(7):315–320
14. American Academy of Pediatric Dentistry (2017) Management of the developing dentition and occlusion in pediatric dentistry. Pediatr Dent 39(6):334–347 456
15. Barberia-Leache E, Suarez-Clua MC, Saavedra-Ontiveros D (2005) Ectopic eruption of the maxillary first permanent molar: characteristics and occurrence in growing children. Angle Orthod 75:610–615
16. Kurol J (2002) Early treatment of tooth-eruption disturbances. Am J Dentofac Orthop 121:588–591
17. Kupietzky A (2000) Correction of ectopic eruption of permanent molars utilizing the brass wire technique. Pediatr Dent 22:408–412
18. Cameron AC, Widmer RP (eds) (2008) Dental anomalies. In: Handbook of pediatric dentistry, 3rd edn. Mosby, London, p 356–357
19. Becker A, Chaushu S (2015) Etiology of maxillary canine impaction: a review. Am J Orthod Dentofac Orthop 148:557–567
20. Liuk IW, Olive RJ, Griffin M et al (2013) Maxillary lateral incisor morphology and palatally displaced canines: a case-controlled cone-beam volumetric tomography study. Am J Orthod Dentofac Orthop 143:522–526
21. Chalakkal P, Thomas AM, Chopra S (2011) Displacement, location, and angulation of unerupted permanent maxillary canines and absence of canine bulge in children. Am J Orthod Dentofac Orthop 139:345–350
22. Bacetti T, Leonardi M, Giuntini V (2010) Distally displaced premolars: a dental anomaly associated with palatally displaced canines. Am J Orthod Dentofac Orthop 138:318–322
23. Bonetti GA, Zanarini M, Parenti SI et al (2011) Preventive treatment of ectopically erupting maxillary permanent canines by extraction of deciduous canines and first molars: a randomized clinical trial. Am J Orthod Dentofac Orthop 139:316–323

24. Tsolakis AI, Kalavritinos M, Bitsanis E (2018) Reliability of different methods for localization of displaced maxillary canines. Am J Orthod Dentofac Orthop 153:308–314
25. Naoumova J, Kurol J, Kjellberg H (2015) Extraction of the deciduous canine as an interceptive treatment in children with palatal displaced canines—part I: shall we extract the deciduous canine or not? Eur J Orthod 37:209–218
26. Schmidt AD, Kokich VG (2007) Periodontal response to early uncovering, autonomous eruption, and orthodontic alignment of palatally impacted maxillary canines. Am J Orthod Dentofac Orthop 131:449–455
27. Neville BW, Damm DD, Allen CM, Chi AC (2016) Abnormalities of teeth. In: Oral and maxillofacial pathology, 4th edn. Elsevier, St. Louis, p 76
28. Shapira Y, Kuftinec MM (2001) Maxillary tooth transpositions: characteristic features and accompanying dental anomalies. Am J Orthod Dentofac Orthop 119:127–134

Anomalies of Tooth Formation

6

6.1 Introduction

The clinical importance of variations of tooth shape and form is seen in many dental disciplines, particularly in pediatric dentistry and orthodontics. Early diagnosis and management of these conditions allows for proper treatment planning, prevents complications in dental development and reduces the need for extensive interventions in the future [1]. Tooth shape is determined during the proliferation and morphogenetic stages of dental development. The interactions between epithelial and mesenchymal tissues during dental development regulate this morphogenesis. To date over 300 genes have been associated with morphogenesis and cell differentiation in teeth [2]. Additionally, the role of the environment and epigenetic factors in tooth formation has still not been clarified [3]. The dental anomalies that occur as a result of these dysregulations are varied and result in an abnormal morphology.

6.2 Pre-eruptive Intracoronal Resorption (PEIR)

6.2.1 Description

Intracoronal radiolucencies found in unerupted teeth were first reported in Skillen in 1941, who used the term "infra-follicular caries" to describe them. Since then, many case reports of this condition have appeared in the dental literature. These defects can resemble dental caries in both clinical and radiographic appearance, thus prompting many authors to refer to them as "pre-eruptive caries" [4]. However, it is unlikely that these radiolucencies represent caries since the tooth is unerupted, covered by dental follicle and therefore not in contact with oral fluids. Histopathologically there is also no evidence of microbial contamination, it is composed of resorptive cells, mostly macrophages and osteoclasts and chronic inflammatory cells [5].

J. A. Soxman et al., *Anomalies of the Developing Dentition*,
https://doi.org/10.1007/978-3-030-03164-0_6

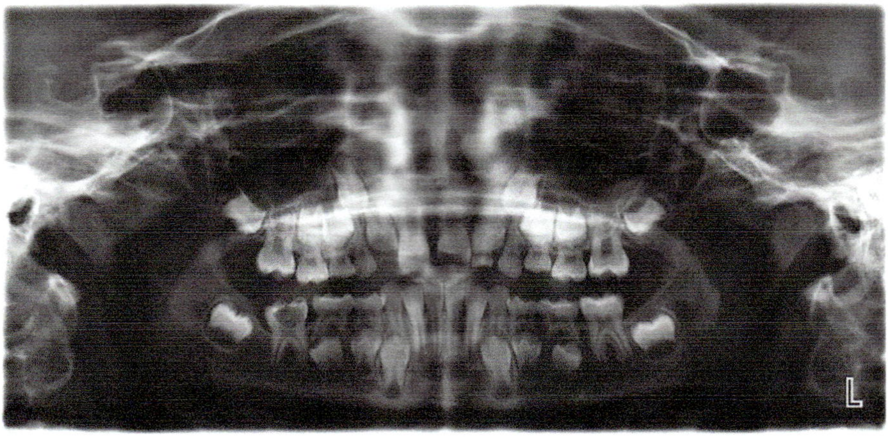

Fig. 6.1 Panormamic radiograph revealing PEIR in unerupted mandibular right permanent first molar

Pre-eruptive intracoronal resorption (PEIR) can only be diagnosed radiographically and it presents as a well-defined radiolucent lesion located in the coronal dentin, just beneath the enamel-dentin junction of unerupted teeth (Fig. 6.1). The condition usually involves a single tooth and more than half of the lesions usually extend less than one third of the width of the thickness of dentin, but this may vary with the stage of presentation [6]. In most cases the overlying enamel is intact. Some lesions progress rapidly, with complete tooth resorption within one to two years and others have a slower progression.

The most frequently involved teeth are the mandibular permanent second molars, mandibular second premolars and third molars. Other teeth reported to have presented with PEIR are permanent first molars and mandibular canines. There are only a few case reports in the primary dentition [4, 7]. The overall prevalence of PEIR is 2–6%, but it varies according to the type of x-ray used to survey and the teeth involved. There are no reported associations with gender, race, medical conditions, systemic factors, or fluoride supplementation [8].

6.2.2 Etiology

The cause of PEIR is not fully understood but the most popular theory is that it is caused by infiltration of resorbtive cells into the dentin while the tooth crown is forming. It is thought that ectopically positioned teeth are predisposed to this condition because of a longer pre-eruptive period. Also, the ectopic eruption of the affected tooth or adjacent tooth can cause a transient or prolonged disruption of tooth formation due to local pressure in area [5].

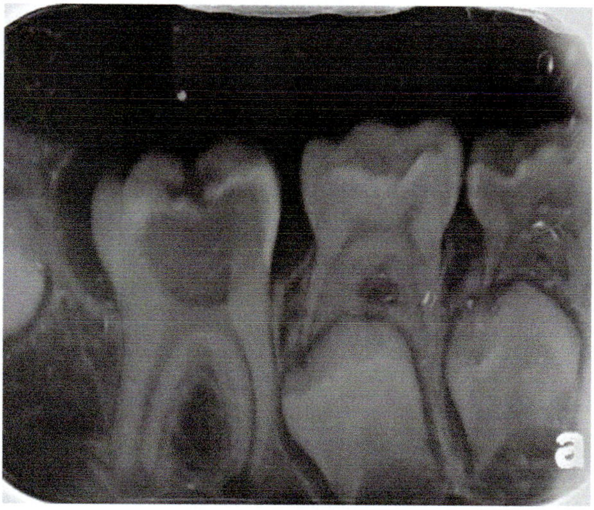

Fig. 6.2 Periapical radiograh revealing a PEIR lesion rapidly progressing and extening into the pulp of mandibular right first permanent molar

6.2.3 Treatment/Management

Some undiagnosed PEIR lesions may progress rapidly, with severe destruction of the dentin crown and endodontic involvement (Fig. 6.2). However, many lesions may enlarge only minimally while in the pre-eruptive stages, so that it may be possible to wait for tooth emergence before restoration [9]. The treatment options discussed in the literature [5] include:

- Surgical exposure and restoration (temporary or permanent) with flap closure of the unerupted tooth as soon as the lesion has been diagnosed radiographically to arrest the progression of the resorptive process and prevent its infiltration into the dental pulp.
- Restoration following eruption and/or monitoring for progression, including pulpal treatment.
- Extraction due to inability to restore

In any case early diagnosis of PEIR is essential to avoid pulp involvement after tooth eruption. Serial radiographs at short intervals could help distinguish between progressive and static lesions and help in treatment decision [10].

6.3 Ectopic Enamel (Enamel Pearl, Cervical Enamel Extension)

6.3.1 Description

Ectopic enamel is present on the roots of teeth as cervical enamel extensions or enamel pearls. Cervical enamel extensions are localized apical projections of the coronal enamel beyond the cervical margin and onto the tooth root. They are flat, triangular, and tapering deposits of enamel that extend apically towards the furcation area. Their reported prevalence ranges from 8.6 to 85% depending on the population studied. The most common location is the buccal surface of mandibular molars. The grading system for cervical enamel extensions grading is from I to III based on their involvement of the furcation. Grade I is just a change in the contour of CEJ with a short extension towards the furcation, Grade II designates when it extends toward the furcation but does not make contact with it and Grade III presence of the extension into the furcation [11]. These deposits can affect plaque removal, complicate scaling and root planing, and may be a local factor in the development of gingivitis and periodontitis. There are strong associations between the presence of cervical enamel extensions and furcation involvement [12]. They also are associated with the formation of an odontogenic inflammatory cyst, the buccal bifurcation cyst [13].

Enamel pearls are ectopic globules of enamel located on the root surface (Fig. 6.3). They were first described in 1842 by Linderer and Linderer as enamel droplets. Other terms used to describe them include enameloma, enamel globule, enamel knot and enamel exostosis. Histologically, enamel pearls can be composed of (1) only enamel, (2) enamel and dentin or (3) enamel, dentin and a pulp horn extending from the coronal pulp chamber or root canal. Their size varies from 0.3 mm to 4 mm, and radiographically appear as well defined radiopaque nodules with a radiodensity similar to enamel adherent to the root surface (Fig. 6.4).

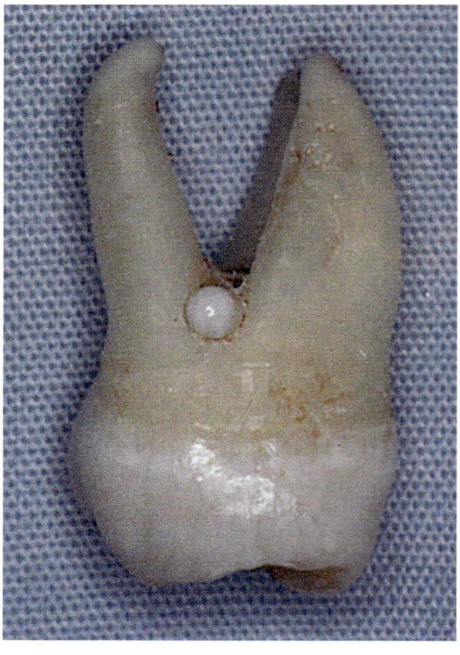

Fig. 6.3 Clinical photograph showing an enamel pearl located in the furcation of an extracted maxillary permanent molar (courtesy of Dr. Carl M. Allen)

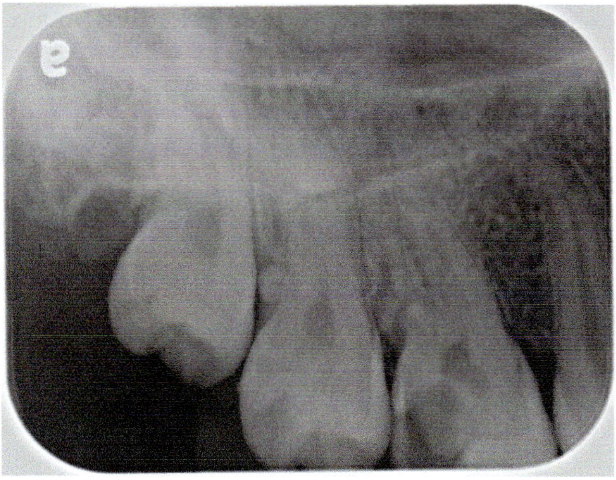

Fig. 6.4 Periapical radiograph revealing enamel pearls on distal surface of maxillary right first and second permanent molars

Only rarely have they been found within dentin and are called internal enamel pearl [14]. They have a distinct preference for the furcation areas of molars, particularly the maxillary third and second molars but they can occur in any area of the root, including apical areas. Their prevalence is 1.1–9.7% [15]. They can present as single or multiple pearls in the same tooth. In 20% of cases, various teeth are involved [16]. The most commonly affected teeth are second and third maxillary molars followed by mandibular molars. Rarely, they have been reported to occur on maxillary premolars, canines, and incisors [17]. Additionally, only few case reports have identified them occurring in primary teeth [18].

6.3.2 Etiology

The etiology of this ectopic enamel is not established, but it theorized that they develop as a result of the localized developmental activity of remnants of Hertwig's epithelial sheath adhered to the root surface. These epithelial cells have the potential to differentiate into ameloblasts and produce the enamel deposits [19].

6.3.3 Treatment/Management

Treatment of cervical enamel extensions is an odontoplasty, or surgical procedure to allow access to proper plaque control by patients to prevent further loss of attachment. Additionally, regenerative procedures may be secondarily necessary to treat the osseous defect created [20].

Enamel pearls can be a risk factor for periodontal disease; since they may compromise connective tissue attachment and may act as reservoirs for periodontal biofilm.

6.4 Dens in Dente (Dens Invaginatus)

6.4.1 Description

Dens in Dente/Dens invaginatus (DI) is a developmental anomaly resulting from invagination of the enamel organ into the dentin papilla before calcification has occurred. The term dens in dente literally means "tooth within a tooth". The first case was described by Tomes in 1859, and later Swanson and McCarthy described the features of DI in depth in their article describing a case of bilateral DI [21]. Two major forms have been described; coronal and radicular. Of these, coronal dens invaginatus is the most common [22].

The most widely used classification system for coronal DI was proposed by Oehlers in 1957 [23] and it classifies them into 3 major types based on radiographic extent of the invagination (Fig. 6.5) [24]. Type I when invagination is minimal, confined to crown of tooth and does not extend beyond cemento-enamel junction (CEJ). Type II when it extends beyond the CEJ but remains in the pulp canal and does not extend into periodontal ligament space. Type IIIA extends into pulp chamber and communicates laterally with periodontal ligament space and Type IIIB extends through root and communicates with PDL through apical foramen. Of these types, the most common is Type I (79%) followed by Type II (15%) and Type III (5%) [25].

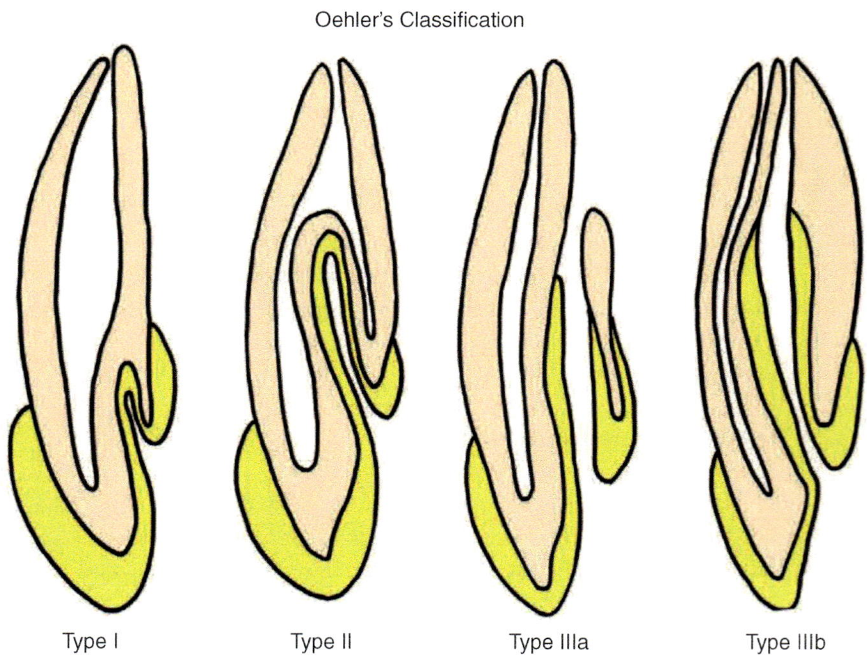

Fig. 6.5 Diagram showing Oehler's Classification System for dens in dente (Reprinted/adapted by permission Springer Nature: Br Dental Journal, Dens invaginatus: diagnosis and management strategies, Gallacher A, Ali R, Bhakta S. 221(7):383–7, 2016)

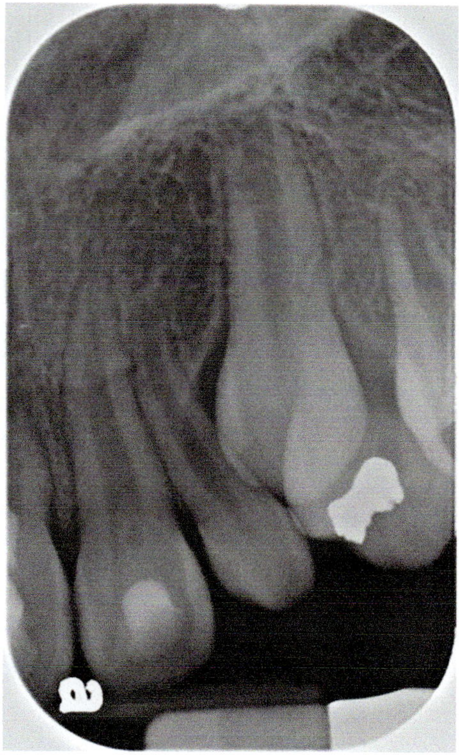

Fig. 6.6 Periapical radiograph revealing a type I dens invaginatus in the maxillary permanent left central incisor

Clinically a tooth with DI may show a deep pit or fissure on the lingual surfaces of anterior teeth, incisal notching or a prominent cingulum. However, a radiographic examination is necessary for the diagnosis of DI. In a periapical x-ray DI appears as a pear-shaped invagination of enamel and dentin with a narrow constriction at the opening on the surface of the tooth (Fig. 6.6). The infolding of the enamel lining is more radiopaque than the surrounding tooth structure and can be therefore easily identified. Rarely, the invagination may be dilated and disturb the normal formation of the tooth resulting in an anomalous tooth. This is the most severe form of DI and for these cases the term dilated odontome is used (Fig. 6.7) [26].

Radicular dens invaginatus is rare and is thought to occur due to an infolding of Hertwig's root sheath with the formation of enamel that extends along the surface of the root. Radiographically the teeth appear to have an enlarged root [27]. The reported prevalence of DI is between 0.3 and 10%. The most commonly affected teeth are permanent maxillary laterals (Fig. 6.8) and it is often bilateral. In decreasing order of frequency, the other teeth that can be affected are central incisors, premolars, canines, and molars [25]. There is a predilection for the maxilla and the occurrence in mandibular teeth is rare with only a few cases reported to date [28]. It has also rarely been reported to occur in primary teeth [29].

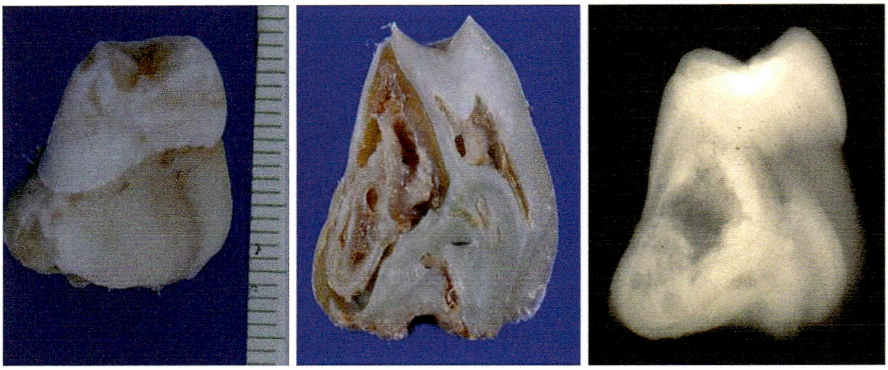

Fig. 6.7 Clinical photographs and radiograph of an extracted maxillary premolar presenting as a dilated odontome, the most severe form of dens invaginatus (courtesy of Dr. Maria A. Copete)

Fig. 6.8 Periapical radograph revealing a type II dens invaginatus in the maxillary left permanent lateral incisor

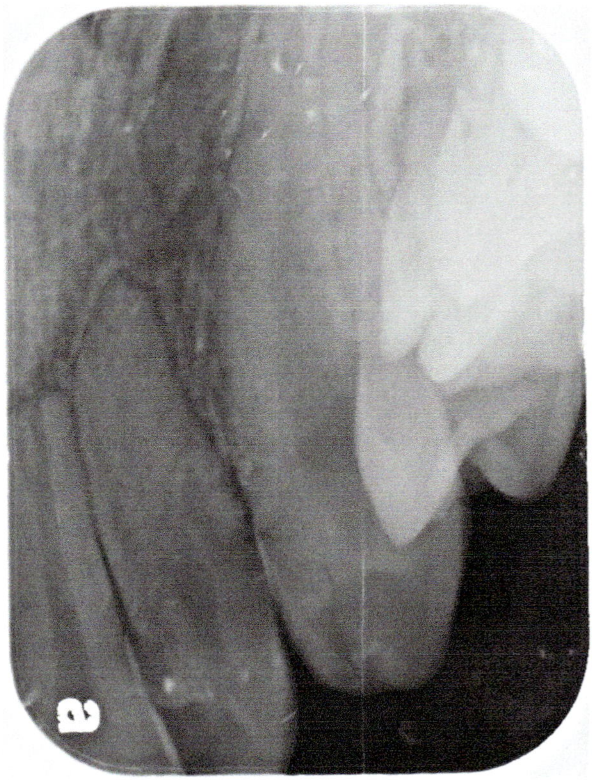

6.4.2 Etiology

The etiology of DI has not been established, but it is likely that genetic factors are involved. Familial clustering has been reported and it tends to occur bilaterally or affect multiple teeth in the same patient. Additionally, patients with evidence of dens invaginatus may also have other dental anomalies such a microdontia (peg lateral), macrodontia, hypodontia and associated syndromes (William's syndrome, Ekman–Westborg–Julin syndrome) [25].

6.4.3 Treatment/Management

Teeth with DI frequently have pulp pathology. Because of the lingual anatomy, it is possible for caries to develop inside the DI without any clinically detectable lesion. Since the enamel lining is thin and close to the pulp chamber, the carious lesion could easily penetrate the pulp chamber. Additionally, there can be thin canals within the enamel of the DI, forming a direct communication with the pulp. The apical periodontium should be examined to check for pulp pathology, and pulp testing should be performed to confirm pulp vitality.

For vital teeth with type I DI, the lingual aspect should be sealed or restored soon after eruption to prevent bacterial communication. For DI type II lesions, removal of carious dentin, placement of calcium hydroxide (CaOH) or mineral trioxide aggregate (MTA) as indirect pulp capping placement of a final restoration is recommended.

For cases with pulp necrosis there is a range of options available to treat them. If the tooth has an open apex, apexification with CaOH or MTA is often successful followed by final obturation. For more complex cases with type III DI endodontic therapy with or without periapical surgery is necessary. Depending on the relationship of the invagination and root canal system, the invagination can either be treated in isolation or in combination with the root canal system if both the pulp and invagination are infected [24]. In cases with large invaginations and abnormal tooth morphology extraction is necessary [30].

6.5 Gemination

6.5.1 Description

Gemination is a dental anomaly that results from the attempt by a single tooth germ to divide. The result is a large single tooth with bifid crown and one root and root canal. Clinically, the tooth count in the arch is normal if the affected tooth is counted as one. Both a clinical and radiographic exam are necessary to make this diagnosis.

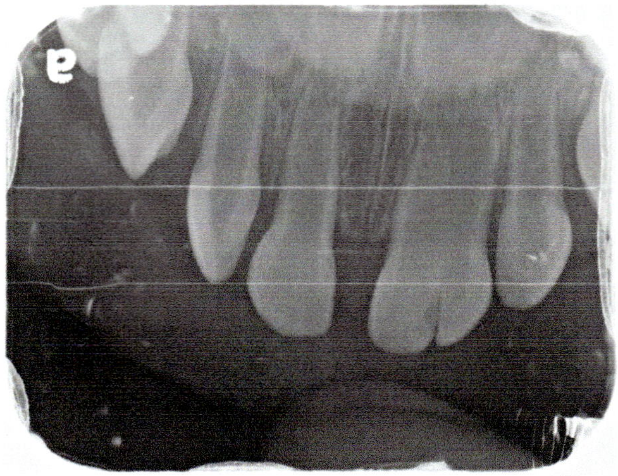

Fig. 6.9 Occlusal radiograph revealing gemination in maxillary primary central incisor. The tooth count in the arch is normal with the geminated incisor counted as one

Geminated teeth are found more frequently in primary dentition than permanent dentition. The prevalence in the permanent dentition is 0.1% and 0.5% in the primary dentition. There is also a higher prevalence in Asian populations. The maxillary central incisors are the teeth most commonly affected by gemination (Fig. 6.9). Geminated teeth are mostly unilateral, and a bilateral presentation is very rare with a prevalence of 0.02% [31].

6.5.2 Etiology

The etiology of gemination is unknown, but trauma causing contact between developing tooth germs, environmental factors, and familial genetic tendency may play a role in their development [32].

6.5.3 Management/Treatment

In the primary dentition gemination can result in crowding, abnormal spacing and can also cause delayed eruption or ectopic eruption of permanent successor (Figs. 6.10 and 6.11). Therefore, early diagnosis is important in order to monitor eruption of the permanent teeth. Extraction may be necessary to allow the permanent tooth to erupt normally. Gemination has not been associated with missing teeth in permanent dentition.

Geminated teeth will result in poor esthetics for the permanent dentition. Crown modification can be attempted. The success of this procedure will be dependent on the amount of tooth that needs to be removed and also on the mesial–distal dimensions at the cemento-enamel junction. Reduction in crown width is possible supragingivally but difficult subgingivally and may lead to periodontal problems [33]. Other options include full crown prosthetic coverage, autotransplantation [34] and in severe cases extraction and replacement of tooth may be necessary [35].

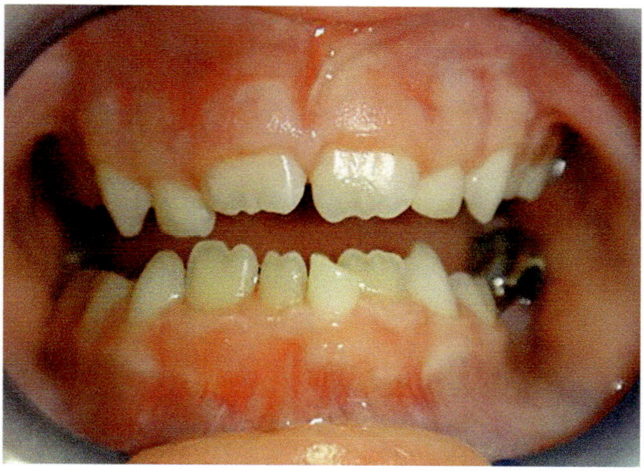

Fig. 6.10 Clinical photograph showing gemination mandibular right permanent central incisor and right and left permanent lateral incisors, agenesis mandibular left permanent central incisor and over-retained primary central incisor

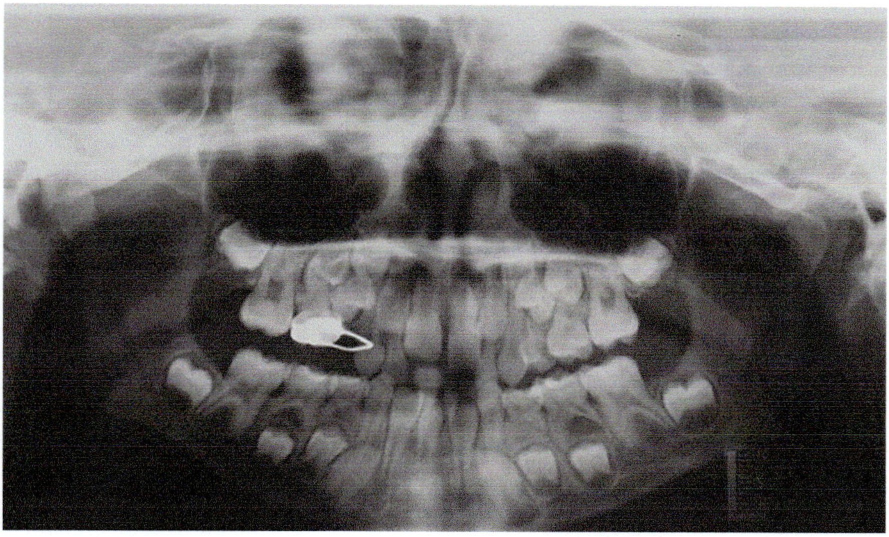

Fig. 6.11 Panoramic radiograph revealing gemination mandibular right permanent central incisor and right and left permanent lateral incisors, agenesis mandibular left permanent central incisor and over-retained primary central incisor

6.6 Fusion

6.6.1 Description

Fusion is a developmental disorder characterized by the union of two adjacent teeth at the crown level (enamel and dentin), causing the formation of a single tooth with an enlarged clinical crown. The tooth count in the arch shows a missing tooth if the abnormal tooth is counted as one. On 0.1% of cases the fusion occurs with a

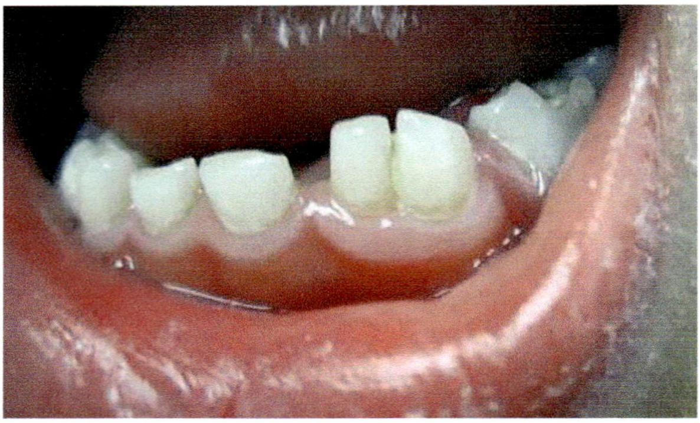

Fig. 6.12 Clinical photograph showing fusion of left primary lateral incisor and canine resulting in a tooth with a bifid crown

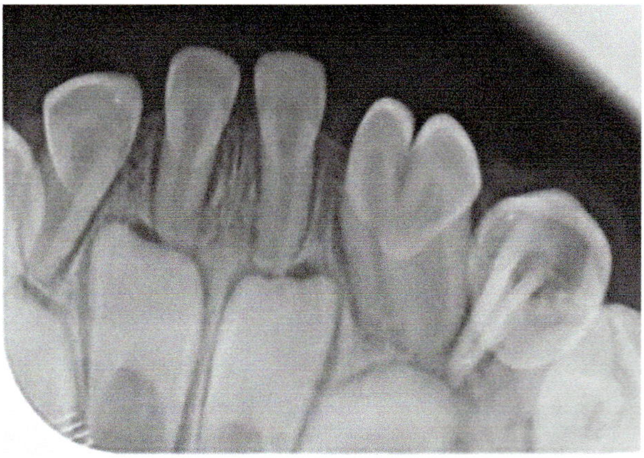

Fig. 6.13 Occlusal radiograph revealing fusion of left primary lateral incisor and canine with two distict root canals

supernumerary tooth, and this is most frequent in the anterior maxilla [36]. In those cases, the tooth count will be normal. Since the differentiation between fusion and gemination can be difficult at times, the term "double teeth" has been used to describe both conditions [37].

A fused tooth is clinically broad and shows either a bifid crown, a groove separating the two crowns or an incisal notch (Fig. 6.12). Most fused teeth show 2 separate roots canals (Fig. 6.13). Bilateral cases are rare with a prevalence of 0.02% [38]. There have also been reports of talon cups associated with fused teeth [39].

Overall the incidence of fusion is approximately 0.1% in the permanent dentition and 0.5% in the primary dentition. In the primary dentition, the most commonly affected teeth are the mandibular lateral incisor and canine or mandibular central incisor and lateral incisor. Fusion in the primary dentition will result in congenital absence or delayed eruption of the permanent successor. Fusion in primary dentition has also been associated with peg shaped (microdont) permanent successor [40]. Other clinical complications associated with fusion are: caries, periodontal disease and compromised esthetics.

6.6.2 Etiology

The etiology of fusion is not fully understood. Some proposed causes include the result of physical forces that put developing teeth in contact or embryological persistence of the interdental lamina between two tooth germs [41].

6.6.3 Management/Treatment

Fusion of teeth usually appears in the anterior region and can cause esthetic problems such as diastema, crowding or dental protrusion. Fused primary teeth are highly correlated with the absence or anomalies of permanent teeth, and the prevalence depends on the combination of fused primary teeth. The combination with the highest probability of permanent tooth microdontia or impaction was maxillary central and lateral incisor, while the highest probability of congenital absence was mandibular lateral incisor and canine [42]. Therefore, fused teeth in the primary dentition require long-term observation until permanent teeth are erupted and in occlusion. Treatment of fused permanent teeth varies greatly and depends on fusion location and extent. Some treatment options include: reshaping of the crown, sectioning and separation into two teeth and restoration, full crown coverage, hemisection and amputation of one root, extraction and replacement or leaving fused teeth untreated [43, 44].

6.7 Concrescence

6.7.1 Description

Concrescence is a developmental anomaly of the teeth in which roots fuse, with no evidence of periodontal space between two or more teeth. The union is below the cemento-enamel junction and affects only cementum (Fig. 6.14). This anomaly may occur between two normal teeth or between a normal tooth and a supernumerary tooth and it may also occur both in erupted or impacted teeth. The amount of union may vary from only a small site to a solid cemental mass along the entire extent of the approximating root surfaces. Concrescence may occur during root formation or after the root is formed. True concrescence occurs during development and acquired concrescence occurs after root formation is complete [45].

The prevalence of concrescence is 0.8% in adult teeth. The literature has not described an age, gender or race predilection. The most frequently affected teeth are located in the posterior maxilla, more commonly the maxillary second and third molars. There are only a few cases reported of concrescence of a third molar and a supernumerary tooth [46]. Concrescence has also rarely been reported to occur in the mandible [45]. Additionally, there are also few reports of concrescence occurring in primary teeth, usually in the anterior maxilla (Fig. 6.15) [47, 48].

Clinically, if erupted, the teeth appear normal. This anomaly can only be diagnosed radiographically. However, it is sometimes difficult to diagnose using plain films.

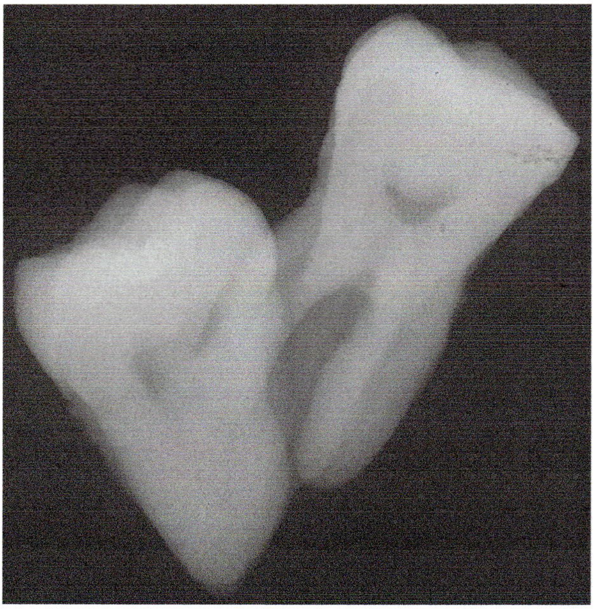

Fig. 6.14 Radiograph showing concrescence of two permanent molars

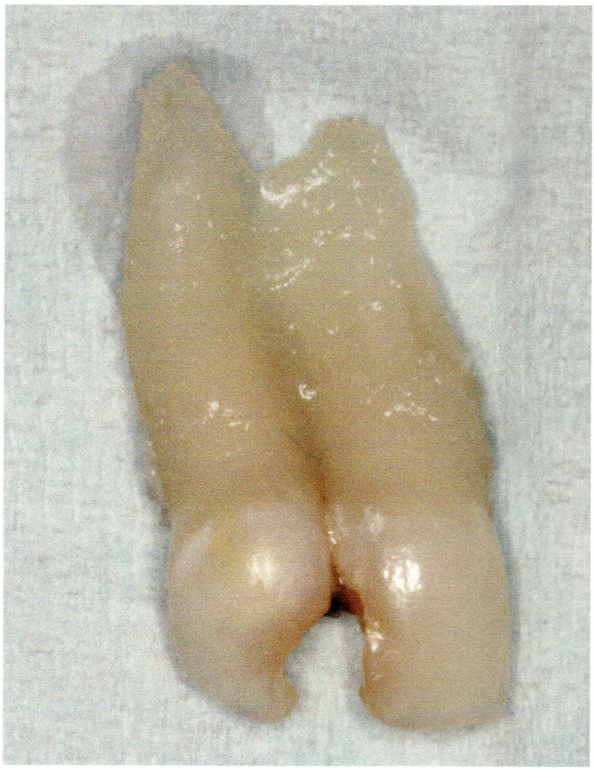

Fig. 6.15 Clinical photograph showing concrescence of two extracted primary incisors, noted only at time of extraction

Therefore, it is important for the clinician to consider the possibility of concrescence when planning extractions when the roots of adjacent teeth are radiographically indistinguishable, especially in the posterior maxilla [49]. The use of cone-beam computer tomography (CBCT) has been proven useful to diagnose this condition [50].

6.7.2 Etiology

Although the exact etiology of concrescence has not yet been explained, space restriction during development, local trauma, excessive occlusal force, or local infection after development may play an important role. All of these lead to interdental bone resorption, allowing the adjacent tooth roots to become fused by the deposition of cementum between them [51].

6.7.3 Treatment

In general, if the concrescence does not affect aesthetics or cause eruption problems, no treatment is necessary. There are case reports of non-surgical root canal treatment done on non-vital teeth with concrescence in order to retain them and maintain natural occlusion [52]. If a tooth extraction is necessary and the anomaly is not detected, surgical complications can occur. The extraction may result in the inadvertent extraction of joined tooth, an alveolar bone fracture, tooth fracture or establishment of an oroantral communication. If a concrescence is suspected before the extraction, it is important that the patient be informed of the condition, the potential complications of the procedure and a surgical plan be established to minimize complications [46, 49].

6.8 Regional Odontodysplasia

6.8.1 Description

Regional odontodysplasia (RO) also known as ghost teeth and it represents a severe nonhereditary developmental disorder of tooth formation that involves epithelial (enamel) and mesenchymal (dentin and cementum) derived dental tissue [53]. The term “odontodysplasia” was introduced by Zegarelli [54] in 1963 as “a rare developmental anomaly involving both mesodermal and ectodermal dental components in a group of contiguous teeth.”

Its prevalence is reported to be less than one in 100,000 and only about 140 cases have been reported in the literature to date. It occurs in both primary and permanent dentitions, and it affects the maxilla twice as frequently as the mandible, with the left maxillary quadrant being the most frequently affected. It is unilateral and it does not cross the midline and the affected teeth are usually contiguous [55]. In the primary maxillary dentition, the most frequently affected teeth are lateral incisors and first and second molars; in the primary mandibular dentition, the most frequently affected tooth is the canine followed by the central and lateral incisors. However, in the in the permanent maxillary dentition, central incisors are most frequently affected, followed by first molars; in the permanent mandibular dentition, the most frequently affected teeth are incisors and canines [56].

The age of the patient at presentation is variable, although it typically manifests during the time of primary tooth eruption or during the mixed dentition. There is a slight female predilection, with a female to male ratio of 1.7–1 [57]. Clinically, the affected teeth have an abnormal morphology and an irregular contour, with superficial pits and grooves and have a yellowish or brownish discoloration (Fig. 6.16). They appear hypoplastic or hypocalcified and the enamel has a softer consistency when probed with an explorer. These teeth are more susceptible to dental caries, and they can fracture by minor trauma [58]. Patients with RO commonly present with delayed, failed, or partial tooth eruption, with or without gingival abscess. In the permanent dentition, teeth usually are not erupted or can be partially erupted with fibrous gingival tissue and swelling.

Radiographically RO shows a lack of contrast between the enamel and dentin. The enamel and dentin are very thin, with only a faint outline seen which gives them a "ghost-like" appearance (Fig. 6.17). The pulp chambers are enlarged, and they have short roots with open apices.

RO is probably misdiagnosed as malformed teeth or odontomas [53]. Primary teeth affected by this anomaly are usually followed by affected permanent successors; however, it is very rare to find normal permanent teeth to follow affected primary teeth.

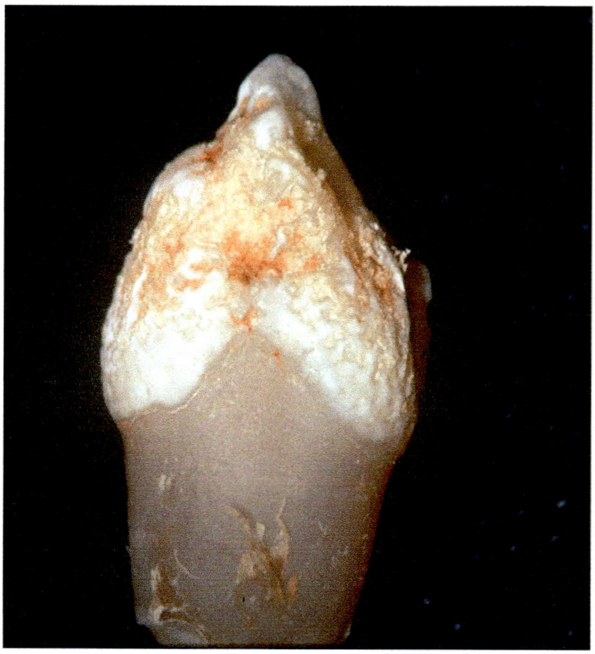

Fig. 6.16 Clinical photograph showing an extracted tooth with regional odontodysplasia with an irregular pitted surface with yellow discoloration (courtesy of Dr. Carl M. Allen)

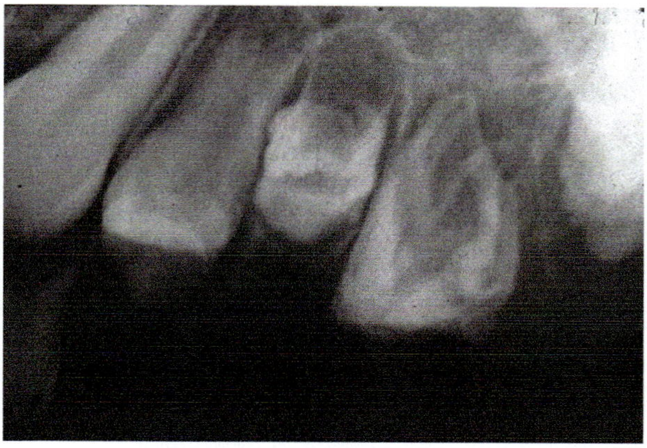

Fig. 6.17 Periapical radiograph of teeth revealing regional odontodysplasia. Described as "ghost teeth" with faint outlines and lack of contrast between enamel and dentin (courtesy of Dr. Carl M. Allen)

6.8.2 Etiology

The etiology of this dental anomaly is unknown. However, various factors have been proposed as the etiologic agents including local trauma or infection, teratogenic medications, local disturbances of the blood supply, Rh incompatibility, radiotherapy, neurologic traumas, fever, metabolic and nutritional disorders and vitamin deficiencies. The most widely accepted theory is an alteration on the vascularization of the affected area, leading to disturbances on tooth development. Heredity seems to play no role in the etiology of this condition because no familial case of such condition has been reported. In addition, RO has been reported in association with some medical conditions such as vascular nevus, hemangiomas, epidermal nevus syndrome, orbital coloboma, facial hypoplasia on the affected side, ectodermal dysplasia, and hydrocephalus [59].

6.8.3 Treatment/Management

A multidisciplinary approach is necessary for the treatment of RO and there is no consensus regarding the treatment. In order to provide a comprehensive treatment plan, factors such as the age of the patient, medical history, previous dental experience, number of affected teeth, and presence or absence of any pathologies should be considered. Some clinicians advocate the removal of affected teeth and use of fixed or removal prosthesis to replace missing teeth. Others advocate for maintaining teeth, except for infected primary teeth, in order to promote normal jaw development. However, in many cases, the prognosis of the affected permanent teeth in RO is poor because of the thin tooth structures, short roots, and open apices. Dental implants are a possible long-term treatment option since the bone quality is not affected in RO [57]. Autotransplantation of teeth has also been reported as treatment option [55].

6.9 Odontoma

6.9.1 Description

Odontomas are developmental defects of dental hard tissues. They have been classified by the World Health Organization as benign, tumor-like odontogenic lesions (hamartoma) [60]. They are composed of all odontogenic tissues (enamel, dentin, cementum and pulp) in varying proportions and in different degrees of development [61]. They can be subdivided into compound and complex odontomas based on their morphology.

In a compound odontoma, the calcified tissue is organized as multiple tooth-like structures or odontoids while in a complex odontoma the calcified mass is amorphous and disorganized [62]. Radiographically compound odontomas appear like multiple well-defined radiopacites surrounded by a slim radiolucent halo (Fig. 6.18). Complex odontomas appear as a well-defined radiopacity with a peripheral radiolucent rim. Occasionally an odontoma can show both compound and complex features. In general, compound odontomas are more common than complex. Compound odontomas have a predilection toward the premaxilla and complex odontomas have a predilection toward the posterior mandible (Fig. 6.19). There is a slight male predilection. In general, odontomas occur more often in the permanent dentition and are very rarely associated with primary teeth [63, 64].

Odontomas typically grow slowly and are asymptomatic. Therefore, they are generally diagnosed by routine radiographic examination in the second and third decades of the life.

Clinically there may be delayed eruption of permanent teeth and less frequently pain and expansion. Rarely odontomas may erupt into the oral cavity [65]. In the early developmental stages of an odontoma in children, calcification is minimal and it may be difficult to diagnose on radiographs. Odontomas can also manifest as part of syndromes, such as Nevus Basal Cell Carcinoma syndrome, Gardner syndrome, familial colonic adenomatosis, Tangier disease or Hermann syndrome [66].

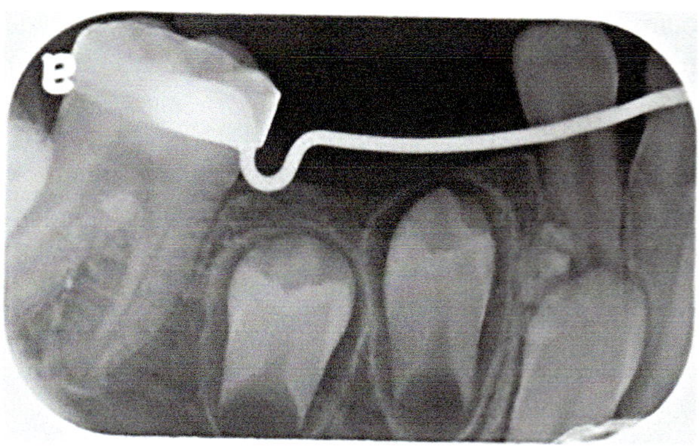

Fig. 6.18 Periapical radiograph of a compound odontoma, revealing multiple tooth-like radiopacities surrounded by radiolucent rim

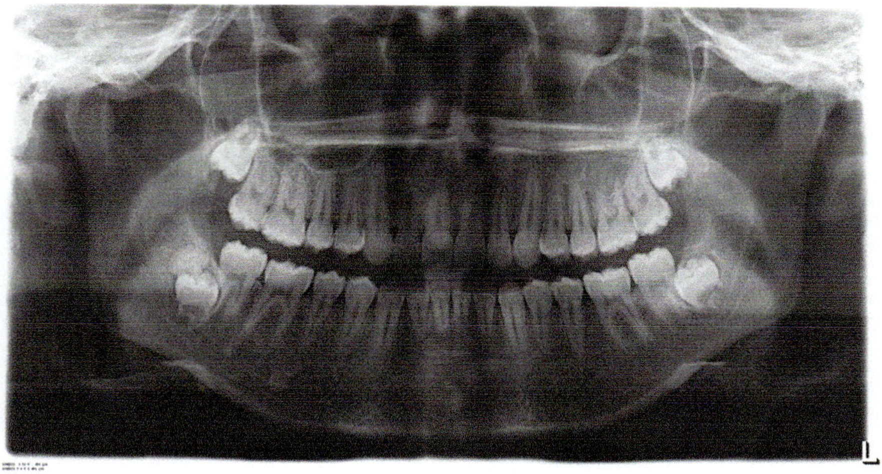

Fig. 6.19 Panoramic radiograph revealing a complex odontoma in right posterior mandible associated with an impacted third molar

6.9.2 Etiology

The etiology of the odontoma is unknown. However, it has been suggested that trauma or infection can induce a growth process in the developing tooth germs. Other probable factors include genetic mutations [67].

6.9.3 Treatment/Management

Treatment consists of complete surgical excision of the lesion. The prognosis is excellent and it does not recur. Histopathologic evaluation of lesion is necessary to confirm the diagnosis and because other odontogenic cysts or tumors may be associated with odontomas, such as dentigerous cyst, calcifying odontogenic cysts, ameloblastic fibroma, and adenomatoid odontogenic tumor (AOT). Early diagnosis and proper treatment is important to allow for normal permanent tooth eruption (Fig. 6.20) [67].

6.10 Molar Root-Incisor Malformation

6.10.1 Description

Molar root-incisor malformation (MRIM) is a newly described dental anomaly affecting the permanent first molars, deciduous second molars, and permanent maxillary central incisors. It was first reported by both Witt [68] and Lee [69] in 2014.

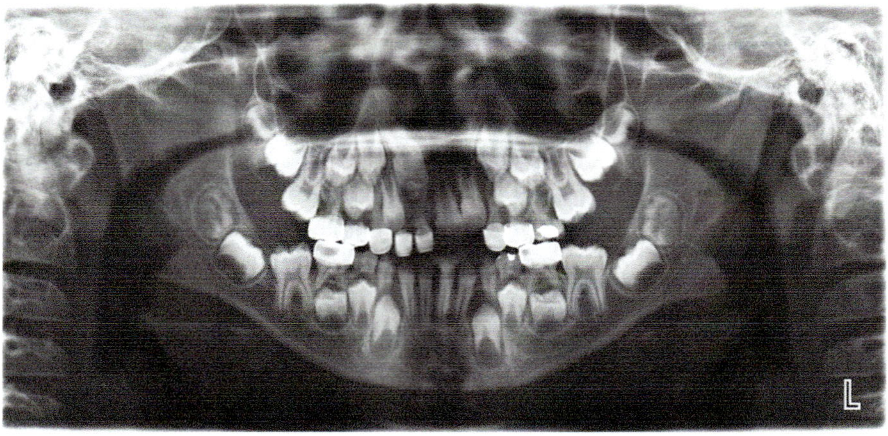

Fig. 6.20 Panoramic radiograph revealing a compound odontoma preventing the eruption of the maxillary right permanent central incisor

Witt et al. described a new developmental root anomaly in two patients with normal crowns and severely dysplastic roots in the first permanent molars. Lee et al. published 12 more patients with this anomaly and used the term Molar Incisor Malformation to describe an anomaly with both molar root malformation and incisor crown defects. Clinically, they found that permanent first molars and deciduous second molars have normal crowns and radiographically have thin, narrow, and short roots, whereas the affected maxillary central incisors can show a hypoplastic enamel notch near the cervical third of the clinical crown.

In 2016 Wright et al. [70] presented 30 new cases and suggested the term Molar root-incisor malformation to help clarify the clinical presentation and avoid confusion with Molar Incisor Hypomineralization, which is an enamel defect. Their results show that the anomaly always affects permanent first molars that show inconspicuous crowns, cervical constriction, dysplastic root formation and diminished pulp chambers (Fig. 6.21). The molar roots are short, tapered and have slit-shaped pulp chambers (Fig. 6.22). This anomaly affects all permanent first molars in a bilateral and symmetric pattern. In contrast, the second primary molars were only affected in 50% cases and maxillary central incisors in 40–58% of cases. Central incisors can show a marked constriction of the crown and an enamel furrow in the cervical third of the crown. This anomaly is detected by radiographic examination or can present as altered or ectopic eruption or as early exfoliation of teeth [71].

6.10.2 Etiology

The etiology of MRIM is thought to involve epigenetic factors related to a systemic disease occurring at around one to two years of age that influence root development. The root morphology is determined by the Hertwig epithelial root sheath that

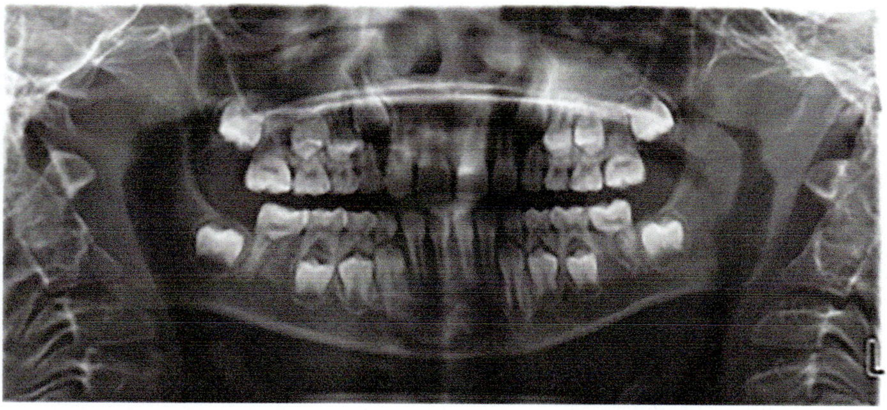

Fig. 6.21 Panoramic radiograph revealing all permanent first molars with molar-root incisor malformation (courtesy of Dr. Bruce Mansbridge)

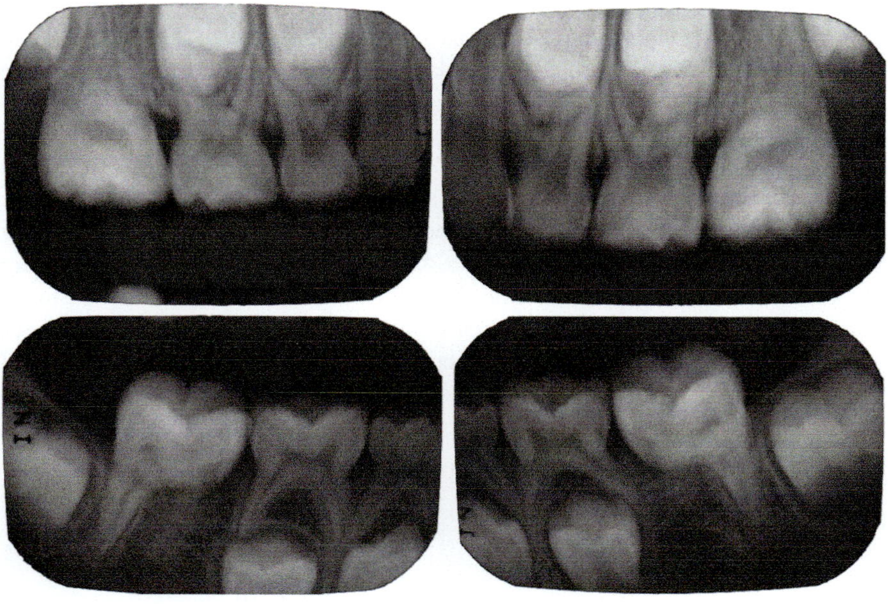

Fig. 6.22 Four periapical radiographs revealing permanent first molars with dysplastic roots and normal clinical crowns, characteristic of molar-root incisor malformation (courtesy of Dr. Bruce Mansbridge)

proliferates from the enamel epithelium at the cemento-enamel junction. Developmental defects in root morphology can result from environmental stressors occurring these critical developmental periods. Most of the MRIM cases reported show severe systemic conditions very early in life suggesting these root malformations are a secondary effect of these systemic stressors. Of the reported cases, the most common stressor or associated abnormality appears to be neurologic [70, 72].

6.10.3 Treatment/Management

Clinical problems associated with MRIM include impaction, early exfoliation, space loss, spontaneous pain, and periapical abscess of the permanent first molar and deciduous second molar. Additionally, the maxillary central incisors affected may have poor esthetics. Therefore, children with a MIM need close follow-up and may require a wider-ranging treatment plan that takes into consideration management of signs and symptoms as well as the long-term prognosis for the teeth involved [73]. The partial root development can complicate orthodontic movement and the furcation abnormality can compromise the periodontal health of the affected teeth.

6.11 Dilaceration

6.11.1 Description

Dilaceration is a term used to describe a malformation occurring during the development of a tooth that disrupts the normal axial relationship between the crown and root of the tooth. It is defined as an angulation or deviation or sharp bend or curve in the linear relationship of the crown of a tooth to its root [74]. The overall incidence of this anomaly is 3.8% [75]. The most frequently affected teeth with root dilaceration are mandibular third molars (24.1%), followed by maxillary first molars (15.3%), maxillary second molars (11.4%), and maxillary third molars (8.1%) [76]. The incidence of dilaceration involving the permanent anterior dentition following trauma to the primary dentition is about 4.7% (Fig. 6.23) [77]. Dilacerations are reported to be a craniofacial manifestation in the following syndromes: Smith-Magenis syndrome, Ehlers-Danlos hypermobility type syndrome, Axenfeld-Rieger syndrome, congenital ichthyosis [78] and Kabuki syndrome (Fig. 6.24) [79]. In

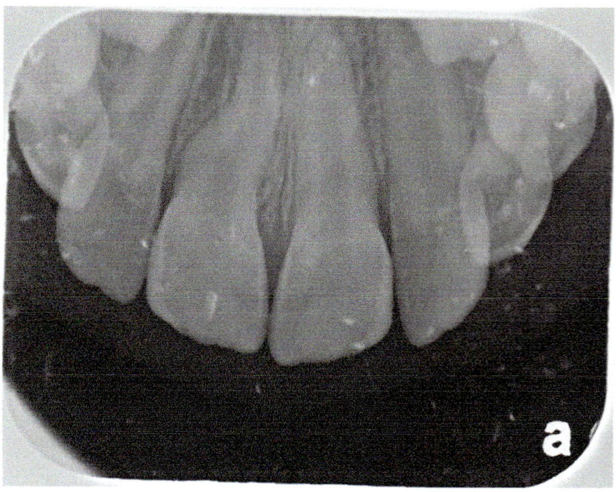

Fig. 6.23 Periapical radiograph revealing dilaceration of the right maxillary permanent central incisor secondary to trauma to primary incisor

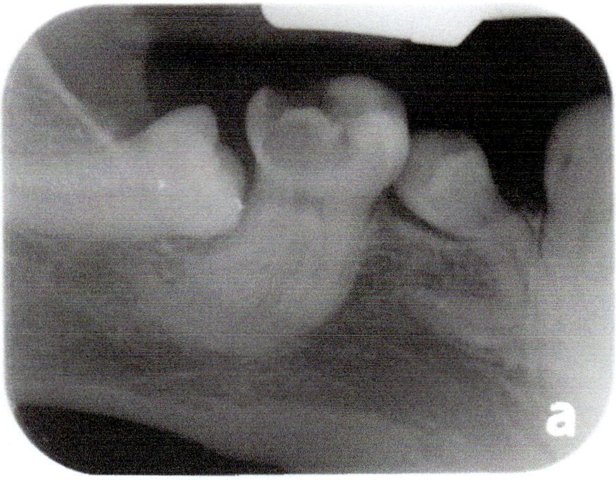

Fig. 6.24 Periapical radiograph revealing severe dilacerations of right mandibular premolar and permanent molar in a patient with Cornelia de Lange syndrome

patients with non-syndromic Cleft Lip/Palate the incidence of anterior tooth dilaceration is not higher than control populations [80].

A periapical radiograph is required to diagnose a dilaceration, but in teeth with curvatures in a vestibular or lingual/palatine direction, a cone beam computer tomography could be of diagnostic utility [81].

Dilacerations are less common in the primary dentition, and usually reported to occur in maxillary incisors and molars [82].

6.11.2 Etiology

When a dilaceration occurs in permanent incisors, it is most often as a result of trauma to the primary predecessors whose apices lie close to the permanent tooth germ. Most injuries to the primary dentition occur between the ages of two and four years by which time the primary teeth have fully formed. An intrusion injury places the apex of the primary tooth in close approximation to the permanent successors developing tooth bud increasing the likelihood of damage to the tooth bud, however, this cannot be the only cause since many cases of dilacerations have no reported history of trauma. Another theory on the etiology is that it is secondary to the ectopic development of the tooth and lack of space since it commonly affects third molars [76].

Other causes involved in the development of a dilaceration are local factors such as the formation of scar tissue, odontogenic infections and the effect of anatomical structures, such as the cortical bone of the sinus, the mandibular canal, and the nasal fossa, which may shift the epithelial diaphragm. Mechanical trauma from orotracheal intubation and laryngoscopy have also been blamed causes for the dilaceration of primary maxillary central incisors as well as the presence of cysts, tumors, odontogenic hamartoma/odontoma (Fig. 6.25), and mechanical interference during the eruption, such as an ankylotic primary tooth the roots of which are non-resorbed [83].

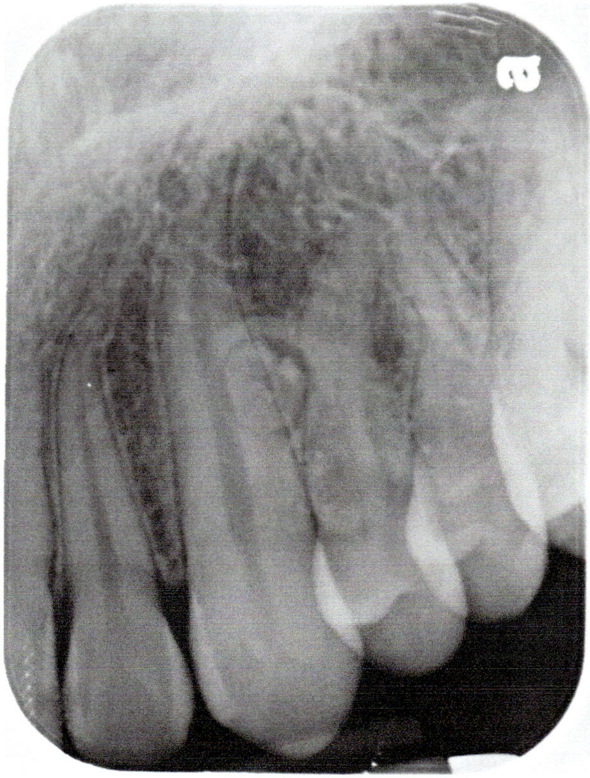

Fig. 6.25 Periapical radiograph revealing a dilaceration of the left maxillary first premolar secondary to an adjacent odontoma

6.11.3 Treatment/Management

Recognizing root dilaceration is vital during root canal treatment because failure to diagnose this condition contributes to a higher rate of endodontic treatment failures. Failure to maintain root canal curvature may result in ledging, apical cavitation, perforation, and instrument breakage. Additionally, dilacerated roots have a higher risk of fracture during tooth extraction. There are also case reports indicating that dilacerated teeth may make orthodontic treatment more complicated [84].

6.12 Short Root Anomaly

6.12.1 Description

Short root anomaly (SRA), also known as root dwarfism or rhizomicry, is a dental anomaly affecting tooth root development characterized by short roots with rounded apices and reduced crown to root ratios. It was first described in the Swedish population by Lind in 1972 [85]. He characterized it objectively as teeth having a root length to crown length ratio of 1.1 or less.

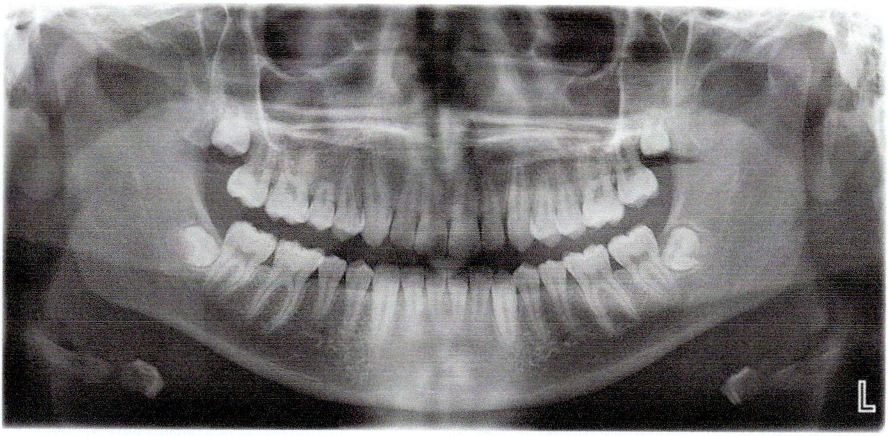

Fig. 6.26 Panoramic radiograph revealing short root anomaly in right maxillary and mandibular second premolars

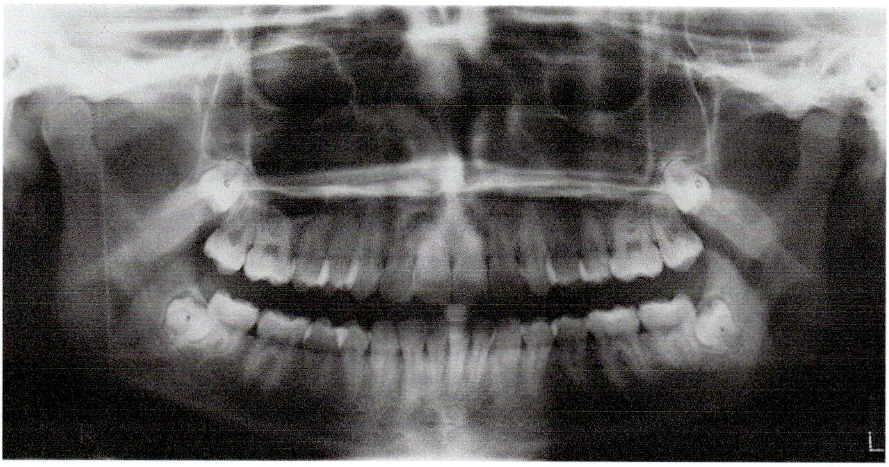

Fig. 6.27 Panoramic radiograph revealing short root anomaly in maxillary permanent central incisors

This disorder affects teeth bilaterally with a predilection for maxillary incisors, and maxillary and mandibular premolars (Figs. 6.26 and 6.27). The mandibular incisors and canines are rarely involved. The apices are rounded rather than pointed. Other dental anomalies including hypodontia, supernumerary teeth, microdontia, dens invaginatus, taurodontism, and obliterated pulp chambers have been reported to occur concurrently (Fig. 6.28) [86]. The reported prevalence in Caucasians is 1.3–2.7%. In the Mongolian and Japanese populations the prevalence is 10%, and there has also been an increasing prevalence reported in the Latino population. A female predilection has been noted and the mean age at diagnosis is14 years of age [87].

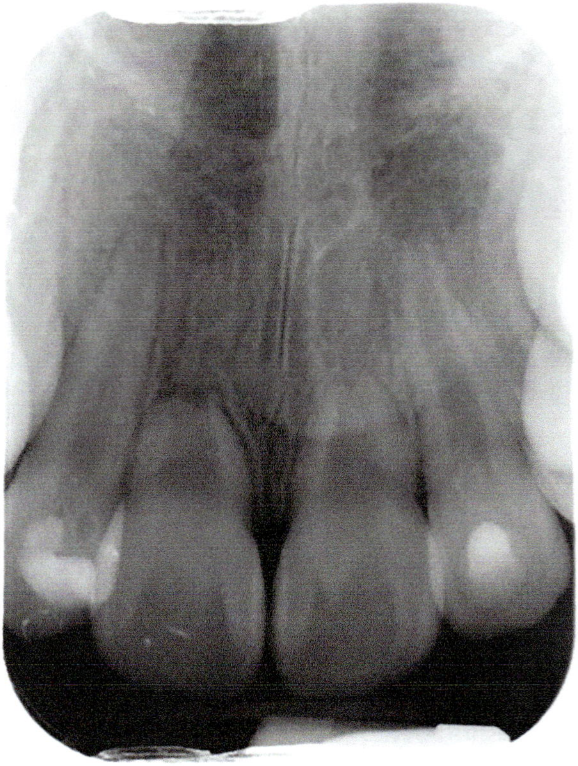

Fig. 6.28 Periapical radiograph revealing maxillary permanent central incisors with short root anomaly and lateral incisors with associated dens in dente

6.12.2 Etiology

The precise etiology of SRA is unknown, although evident familial clustering suggests that a genetic component at least plays a role. An autosomal dominant inheritance pattern has been documented [88]. Since the affected roots lack any signs of hard tissue resorption, this would indicate that the processes of root morphogenesis occurs normally, but the root growth in length; that is the apical growth of HERS (Hertwig epithelial root sheath) is deficient. Additionally, the expression of matrix metalloproteinases (MMPs) in the gingival crevicular fluid of patients with SRA, was studied and there was no significant resorptive or pathological activity in the crevicular fluid of the affected teeth further supporting the conclusion that it is a developmental condition [89].

6.12.3 Treatment/Management

The prevalence of misdiagnosis of SRA is a significant concern given its influence on treatment planning, especially for orthodontics. There is evidence that unusual root morphology before orthodontic treatment can increase the risk of root resorption. Specifically, patients with SRA have an increased risk of root resorption during orthodontic treatment [90]. Therefore, it is important to detect the condition in patients at the pre-treatment stage and carefully plan orthodontic treatment. This highlights the importance of a proper pretreatment radiographic examination, particularly periapical radiographs of the incisors, which have a higher predilection for SRA. As far as orthodontic treatment, careful mechanics and minimal orthodontic forces are required for successful maintenance of root/crown ratio in patients with SRA [91].

6.13 Accessory Roots (Supernumerary Roots)

6.13.1 Description

An accessory or supernumerary root is the development of an additional root in a tooth that is not part of the normal anatomy. It can occur both in the primary and permanent dentition. In the permanent dentition, supernumerary roots are not uncommon, with single-rooted permanent premolars and canines being more frequently affected (Fig. 6.29) [92]. Rarely maxillary anterior teeth can present with an additional root [93].

The prevalence of increased root number is less common in the primary dentition than in the permanent [94]. Maxillary canines and mandibular molars are more frequently affected, compared to mandibular canines and maxillary molars [95]. The prevalence of bi-rooted primary canines appears to be higher in the maxilla (Fig. 6.30) than the mandible and more case reports are published in Asian populations that Caucasians, suggesting a racial predilection [96].

Maxillary molars with four roots and mandibular molars with three roots are also noted. The term radix entomolares is used to describe a distolingual supernumerary root on a mandibular first molar (Fig. 6.31). The frequency varies among different

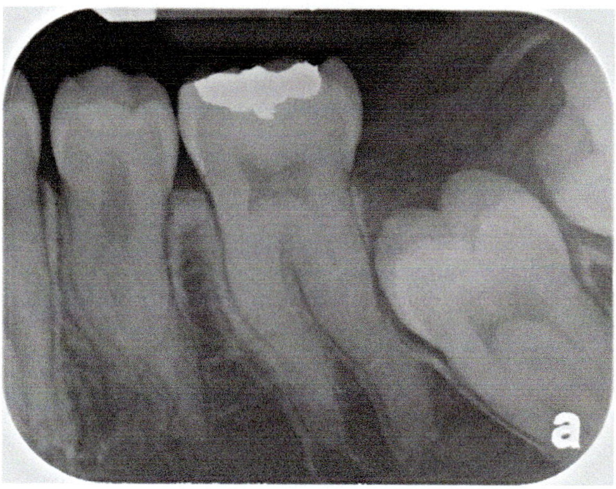

Fig. 6.29 Periapical radiograph revealing a supernumerary root in the left mandibular second premolar

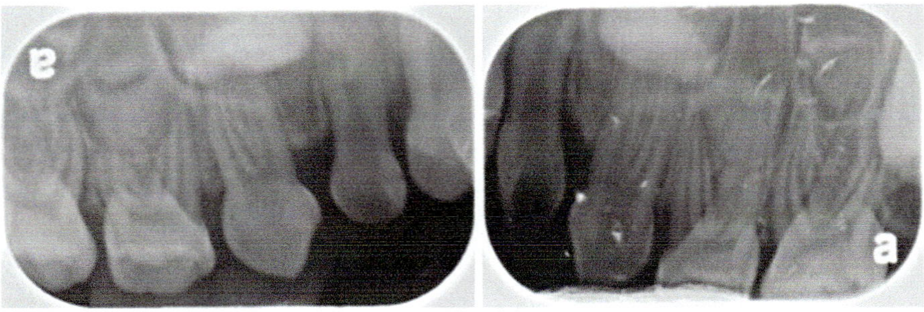

Fig. 6.30 Two periapical radiographs of the same patient revealing bilateral bi-rooted maxillary primary canines

Fig. 6.31 Periapical radiograph revealing radix entomolaris; a supernumerary distolingual root on left mandibular first permanent molar and a supernumerary root on left mandibular second molar

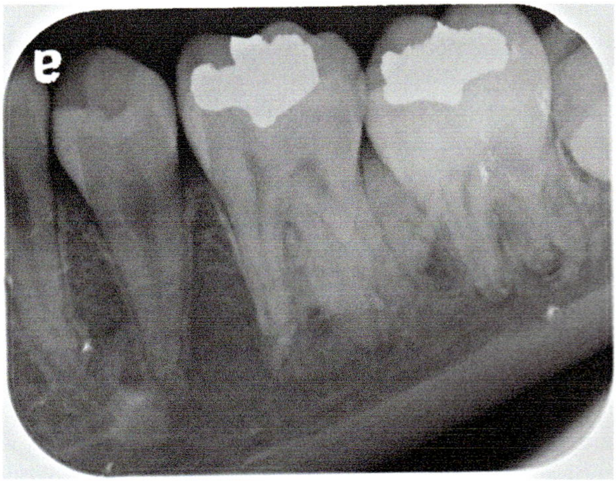

ethnicities. In races of Asian origin including Malay, Chinese, Japanese, Inuit, and Native American it can be seen in 8–43% in contrast to only 3.2–4.2% of Caucasians and 0.65–2.85% of Blacks. In primary molars, a prevalence of 0.67–27.8% is reported, depending on the population studied [97].

6.13.2 Etiology

Accessory roots are thought to be caused by but traumatic injuries to Hertwig's epithelial root sheath during root formation, or by genetic factors [98]. The formation of an accessory root usually occurs through either splitting the Hertwig's epithelial root sheath (HERS) to form two similar roots or by folding of the HERS to create an independent root which may have various morphological features [99].

6.13.3 Treatment/Management

Thorough knowledge of both root and root canal morphology is fundamental for successful root canal treatment. Frequently, root canals are left untreated because the clinicians fail to identify their presence. Close evaluation of pre-operative radiographs is necessary and in some instances, may require further imagining with cone beam computer tomography to establish the presence of an additional root.

Unrecognized anomalies of primary root morphology may lead to clinical difficulties with endodontic treatment or extractions. With multi-rooted primary teeth, interference with the normal development of the permanent dentition can occur, and therefore should be monitored. Difficulties in resorption of the primary tooth and abnormal eruption path of the permanent successor may also occur [96].

References

1. Brook AH, Jernvall J, Smith RN, Hughes TE, Townsend GC (2014) The dentition: the outcomes of morphogenesis leading to variations of tooth number, size and shape. Aust Dent J 59(Suppl 1):131–142
2. Thesleff I (2006) The genetic basis of tooth development and dental defects. Am J Med Genet A 140(23):2530–2535
3. Townsend G, Bockmann M, Hughes T, Brook A (2012) Genetic, environmental and epigenetic influences on variation in human tooth number, size and shape. Odontology 100(1):1–9
4. Seow WK, Hackley D (1996) Pre-eruptive resorption of dentin in the primary and permanent dentitions: case reports and literature review. Pediatr Dent 18(1):67–71
5. Wong L, Khan S (2014) Occult caries or pre-eruptive intracoronal resorption? A chance finding on a radiograph. Pediatr Dent 36(5):429–432
6. Manmontri C, Chompu-Inwai P, Mahasantipiya PM, Prapayasatok S (2018) Prevalence of pre-eruptive intracoronal radiolucencies in Thai children and adolescents: a retrospective study. J Investig Clin Dent 9(2):e12303
7. Schwimmer Y, Zeltser R, Moskovitz M (2017) Deep caries due to Pre-eruptive intracoronal resorption in a newly erupted primary molar. Int J Paediatr Dent 27(4):313–315
8. Davidovich E, Kreiner B, Peretz B (2005) Treatment of severe pre-eruptive intracoronal resorption of a permanent second molar. Pediatr Dent 27(1):74–77
9. Seow WK (2000) Pre-eruptive intracoronal resorption as an entity of occult caries. Pediatr Dent 22(5):370–376
10. Moskovitz M, Holan G (2004) Pre-eruptive intracoronal radiolucent defect: a case of a nonprogressive lesion. J Dent Child (Chic) 71(2):175–178
11. Chan HL, Oh TJ, Bashutski J, Fu JH, Wang HL (2010) Cervical enamel projections in unusual locations: a case report and mini-review. J Periodontol 81(5):789–795
12. Attar NB, Phadnaik MB (2009) Bilateral cervicoenamel projection and its management: a case report with lingual involvement. J Indian Soc Periodontol 13(3):168–171
13. Ramos LM, Vargas PA, Coletta RD, de Almeida OP, Lopes MA (2012) Bilateral buccal bifurcation cyst: case report and literature review. Head Neck Pathol 6(4):455–459
14. Kaugars GE (1983) Internal enamel pearls: report of case. J Am Dent Assoc 107(6):941–943
15. Akgul N, Caglayan F, Durna N, Sumbullu MA, Akgul HM, Durna D (2012) Evaluation of enamel pearls by cone-beam computed tomography (CBCT). Med Oral Patol Oral Cir Bucal 17(2):e218–e222

16. Darwazeh A, Hamasha AA (2000) Radiographic evidence of enamel pearls in jordanian dental patients. Oral Surg Oral Med Oral Pathol Oral Radiol Endod 89(2):255–258
17. Moskow BS, Canut PM (1990) Studies on root enamel (2). Enamel pearls. A review of their morphology, localization, nomenclature, occurrence, classification, histogenesis and incidence. J Clin Periodontol 17(5):275–281
18. Kupietzky A, Rozenfarb N (1993) Enamel pearls in the primary dentition: report of two cases. ASDC J Dent Child 60(1):63–66
19. Versiani MA, Cristescu RC, Saquy PC, Pecora JD, de Sousa-Neto MD (2013) Enamel pearls in permanent dentition: case report and micro-CT evaluation. Dentomaxillofac Radiol 42(6):20120332
20. Zenobio EG, Vieira TR, Bustamante RP, Gomes HE, Shibli JA, Soares RV (2015) Enamel pearls implications on periodontal disease. Case Rep Dent 2015:236462
21. Swanson WF, McCarthy CF Jr (1947) Bilateral dens in dente. J Dent Res 26(2):167–171
22. Hulsmann M (1997) Dens invaginatus: aetiology, classification, prevalence, diagnosis, and treatment considerations. Int Endod J 30(2):79–90
23. Oehlers FA (1957) Dens invaginatus (dilated composite odontome). II Associated posterior crown forms and pathogenesis. Oral Surg Oral Med Oral Pathol 10(12):1302–1316
24. Gallacher A, Ali R, Bhakta S (2016) Dens invaginatus: diagnosis and management strategies. Br Dent J 221(7):383–387
25. Alani A, Bishop K (2008) Dens invaginatus. Part 1: classification, prevalence and aetiology. Int Endod J 41(12):1123–1136
26. Cukovic-Bagic I, Macan D, Dumancic J, Manojlovic S, Hat J (2010) Dilated odontome in the mandibular third molar region. Oral Surg Oral Med Oral Pathol Oral Radiol Endod 109(2):e109–e113
27. Payne M, Craig GT (1990) A radicular dens invaginatus. Br Dent J 169(3-4):94–95
28. Agrawal PK, Wankhade J, Warhadpande M (2016) A rare case of type III dens invaginatus in a mandibular second premolar and its nonsurgical endodontic management by using cone-beam computed tomography: a case report. J Endod 42(4):669–672
29. Barbosa Brandao EC, Aguiar Ribeiro A, Alto Seabra LM (2017) Rare condition of dens invaginatus in a maxillary primary molar and a birooted maxillary primary canine diagnosed during routine examination. Int J Clin Pediatr Dent 10(2):193–195
30. Bishop K, Alani A (2008) Dens invaginatus. Part 2: clinical, radiographic features and management options. Int Endod J 41(12):1137–1154
31. Duncan WK, Helpin ML (1987) Bilateral fusion and gemination: a literature analysis and case report. Oral Surg Oral Med Oral Pathol 64(1):82–87
32. Schuurs AH, van Loveren C (2000) Double teeth: review of the literature. ASDC J Dent Child 67(5):313–325
33. Shah P, Chander JM, Noar J, Ashley PF (2012) Management of 'double teeth' in children and adolescents. Int J Paediatr Dent 22(6):419–426
34. Spuller RL, Harrington M (1986) Gemination of a maxillary permanent central incisor treated by autogenous transplantation of a supernumerary incisor: case report. Pediatr Dent 8(4):299–302
35. Finkelstein T, Shapira Y, Bechor N, Shpack N (2015) Fused and geminated permanent maxillary central incisors: prevalence, treatment options, and outcome in orthodontic patients. J Dent Child (Chic) 82(3):147–152
36. Croll TP, Rains NJ, Chen E (1981) Fusion and gemination in one dental arch: report of case. ASDC J Dent Child 48(4):297–299
37. Aguilo L, Gandia JL, Cibrian R, Catala M (1999) Primary double teeth. A retrospective clinical study of their morphological characteristics and associated anomalies. Int J Paediatr Dent 9(3):175–183
38. Tomizawa M, Shimizu A, Hayashi S, Noda T (2002) Bilateral maxillary fused primary incisors accompanied by succedaneous supernumerary teeth: report of a case. Int J Paediatr Dent 12(3):223–227

39. Danesh G, Schrijnemakers T, Lippold C, Schafer E (2007) A fused maxillary central incisor with dens evaginatus as a talon cusp. Angle Orthod 77(1):176–180
40. Yuen SW, Chan JC, Wei SH (1987) Double primary teeth and their relationship with the permanent successors: a radiographic study of 376 cases. Pediatr Dent 9(1):42–48
41. de Siqueira VC, Braga TL, Martins MA, Raitz R, Martins MD (2004) Dental fusion and dens evaginatus in the permanent dentition: literature review and clinical case report with conservative treatment. J Dent Child (Chic) 71(1):69–72
42. Tsujino K, Yonezu T, Shintani S (2013) Effects of different combinations of fused primary teeth on eruption of the permanent successors. Pediatr Dent 35(2):E64–E67
43. Karacay S, Guven G, Koymen R (2006) Management of a fused central incisor in association with a macrodont lateral incisor: a case report. Pediatr Dent 28(4):336–340
44. Tuna E, Yildirim M, Seymen F, Gencay K, Ozgen M (2009) Fused teeth: a review of the treatment options. J Dent Child (Chic) 76(2):109–116
45. Gunduz K, Sumer M, Sumer AP, Gunhan O (2006) Concrescence of a mandibular third molar and a supernumerary fourth molar: report of a rare case. Br Dent J 200(3):141–142
46. Romito LM (2004) Concrescence: report of a rare case. Oral Surg Oral Med Oral Pathol Oral Radiol Endod 97(3):325–327
47. Sharma U, Gulati A, Gill NC (2013) Concrescent triplets involving primary anterior teeth. Contemp Clin Dent 4(1):94–96
48. Singh A, Bhatia HP, Sharma N (2017) Coexistence of fusion and concrescence of primary teeth: in a child with Down syndrome. Spec Care Dentist 37(3):147–149
49. Palermo D, Davies-House A (2016) Unusual finding of concrescence. BMJ Case Rep 2016:bcr2016214597
50. Syed AZ, Alluri LC, Mallela D, Frazee T (2016) Concrescence: cone-beam computed tomography imaging perspective. Case Rep Dent 2016:8597872
51. Sugiyama M, Ogawa I, Suei Y, Tohmori H, Higashikawa K, Kamata N (2007) Concrescence of teeth: cemental union between the crown of an impacted tooth and the roots of an erupted tooth. J Oral Pathol Med 36(1):60–62
52. Foran D, Komabayashi T, Lin LM (2012) Concrescence of permanent maxillary second and third molars: case report of non-surgical root canal treatment. J Oral Sci 54(1):133–136
53. Matsuyama J, Tanaka R, Iizawa F, Sano T, Kinoshita-Kawano S, Hayashi-Sakai S, Mitomi T (2014) Clinical and radiographic findings and usefulness of computed tomographic assessment in two children with regional odontodysplasia. Case Rep Dent 2014:764393
54. Zegarelli EV, Kutscher AH, Applebaum E, Archard HO (1963) Odontodysplasia. Oral Surg Oral Med Oral Pathol 16:187–193
55. Ziegler S, Neukam FW (2012) Regional odontodysplasia: orthodontic treatment and transplantation of premolars. Am J Orthod Dentofac Orthop 142(5):710–719
56. Al-Tuwirqi A, Lambie D, Seow WK (2014) Regional odontodysplasia: literature review and report of an unusual case located in the mandible. Pediatr Dent 36(1):62–67
57. Hamdan MA, Sawair FA, Rajab LD, Hamdan AM, Al-Omari IK (2004) Regional odontodysplasia: a review of the literature and report of a case. Int J Paediatr Dent 14(5):363–370
58. Rashidian A, Afsharian Zadeh M, Azarshab M, Zarrabian T (2013) Regional odontodysplasia: report of a case. J Dent (Shiraz) 14(4):197–200
59. Carlos R, Contreras-Vidaurre E, Almeida O, Silva K, Abrahão P, Miranda A, Pires F (2008) Regional odontodysplasia: morphological, ultrastructural, and immunohistochemical features of the affected teeth, connective tissue, and odontogenic remnants. J Dent Child (Chic) 75(2):144–150
60. Tuczynska A, Bartosik D, Abu-Fillat Y, Soltysik A, Matthews-Brzozowska T (2015) Compound odontoma in the mandible—case study and literature review. Dev Period Med 19(4):484–489
61. Pippi R (2014) Odontomas and supernumerary teeth: is there a common origin? Int J Med Sci 11(12):1282–1297
62. Yeung KH, Cheung RC, Tsang MM (2003) Compound odontoma associated with an unerupted and dilacerated maxillary primary central incisor in a young patient. Int J Paediatr Dent 13(3):208–212

63. Altay MA, Ozgur B, Cehreli ZC (2016) Management of a compound odontoma in the primary dentition. J Dent Child (Chic) 83(2):98–101
64. Noonan RG (1971) A compound odontoma associated with a deciduous tooth. Oral Surg Oral Med Oral Pathol 32(5):740–742
65. Serra-Serra G, Berini-Aytes L, Gay-Escoda C (2009) Erupted odontomas: a report of three cases and review of the literature. Med Oral Patol Oral Cir Bucal 14(6):E299–E303
66. Hidalgo-Sanchez O, Leco-Berrocal MI, Martinez-Gonzalez JM (2008) Metaanalysis of the epidemiology and clinical manifestations of odontomas. Med Oral Patol Oral Cir Bucal 13(11):E730–E734
67. Kalra A, Sheehy EC, Johnson J, McDonald F (2018) A bag of marbles: a fascinating compound odontoma of the maxilla. Pediatr Dent 40(2):140–142
68. Witt CV, Hirt T, Rutz G, Luder HU (2014) Root malformation associated with a cervical mineralized diaphragm—a distinct form of tooth abnormality? Oral Surg Oral Med Oral Pathol Oral Radiol 117(4):e311–e319
69. Lee HS, Kim SH, Kim SO, Lee JH, Choi HJ, Jung HS, Song JS (2014) A new type of dental anomaly: molar-incisor malformation (MIM). Oral Surg Oral Med Oral Pathol Oral Radiol 118(1):101–9.e3
70. Wright JT, Curran A, Kim KJ, Yang YM, Nam SH, Shin TJ, Hyun HK, Kim YJ, Lee SH, Kim JW (2016) Molar root-incisor malformation: considerations of diverse developmental and etiologic factors. Oral Surg Oral Med Oral Pathol Oral Radiol 121(2):164–172
71. McCreedy C, Robbins H, Newell A, Mallya SM (2016) Molar-incisor malformation: two cases of a newly described dental anomaly. J Dent Child (Chic) 83(1):33–37
72. Lee HS, Kim SH, Kim SO, Choi BJ, Cho SW, Park W, Song JS (2015) Microscopic analysis of molar—incisor malformation. Oral Surg Oral Med Oral Pathol Oral Radiol 119(5):544–552
73. Brusevold IJ, Bie TMG, Baumgartner CS, Das R, Espelid I (2017) Molar incisor malformation in six cases: description and diagnostic protocol. Oral Surg Oral Med Oral Pathol Oral Radiol 124(1):52–61
74. Topouzelis N, Tsaousoglou P, Gofa A (2010) Management of root dilaceration of an impacted maxillary central incisor following orthodontic treatment: an unusual therapeutic outcome. Dent Traumatol 26(6):521–526
75. Hamasha AA, Al-Khateeb T, Darwazeh A (2002) Prevalence of dilaceration in Jordanian adults. Int Endod J 35(11):910–912
76. Malcic A, Jukic S, Brzovic V, Miletic I, Pelivan I, Anic I (2006) Prevalence of root dilaceration in adult dental patients in Croatia. Oral Surg Oral Med Oral Pathol Oral Radiol Endod 102(1):104–109
77. Ben-Bassat Y, Brin I, Zilberman Y (1989) Effects of trauma to the primary incisors on their permanent successors: multidisciplinary treatment. ASDC J Dent Child 56(2):112–116
78. Spoerri A, Signorelli C, van Waes H (2015) Surgical repositioning of a developing maxillary central incisor. A case report. Int J Paediatr Dent 25(4):305–308
79. do Prado Sobral S, Leite AF, Figueiredo PT, Ferrari I, Safatle HP, Cordoba MS, Versiani BR, Acevedo AC, Mestrinho HD (2013) Craniofacial and dental features in kabuki syndrome patients. Cleft Palate Craniofac J 50(4):440–447
80. Weckwerth GM, Santos CF, Brozoski DT, Centurion BS, Pagin O, Lauris JR, Carvalho IM, Neves LT (2016) Taurodontism, root dilaceration, and tooth transposition: a radiographic study of a population with nonsyndromic cleft lip and/or palate. Cleft Palate Craniofac J 53(4):404–412
81. Fuentes R, Farfan C, Astete N, Navarro P, Arias A (2018) Distal root curvatures in mandibular molars: analysis using digital panoramic X-rays. Folia Morphol (Warsz) 77(1):131–137
82. Kilpatrick NM, Hardman PJ, Welbury RR (1991) Dilaceration of a primary tooth. Int J Paediatr Dent 1(3):151–153
83. Topouzelis N, Tsaousoglou P, Pisoka V, Zouloumis L (2010) Dilaceration of maxillary central incisor: a literature review. Dent Traumatol 26(5):427–433

84. Tanaka E, Hasegawa T, Hanaoka K, Yoneno K, Matsumoto E, Dalla-Bona D, Yamano E, Suekawa Y, Watanabe M, Tanne K (2006) Severe crowding and a dilacerated maxillary central incisor in an adolescent. Angle Orthod 76(3):510–518
85. Lind V (1972) Short root anomaly. Scand J Dent Res 80(2):85–93
86. Desai RS, Vanaki SS, Puranik RS, Rashmi GS, Nidawani P (2006) An unusual combination of idiopathic generalized short-root anomaly associated with microdontia, taurodontia, multiple dens invaginatus, obliterated pulp chambers and infected cyst: a case report. J Oral Pathol Med 35(7):407–409
87. Puranik CP, Hill A, Henderson Jeffries K, Harrell SN, Taylor RW, Frazier-Bowers SA (2015) Characterization of short root anomaly in a Mexican cohort—hereditary idiopathic root malformation. Orthod Craniofac Res 18(Suppl 1):62–70
88. Apajalahti S, Arte S, Pirinen S (1999) Short root anomaly in families and its association with other dental anomalies. Eur J Oral Sci 107(2):97–101
89. Apajalahti S, Sorsa T, Ingman T (2003) Matrix metalloproteinase -2, -8, -9, and -13 in gingival crevicular fluid of short root anomaly patients. Eur J Orthod 25(4):365–369
90. Marques LS, Generoso R, Armond MC, Pazzini CA (2010) Short-root anomaly in an orthodontic patient. Am J Orthod Dentofac Orthop 138(3):346–348
91. Dutra EH, Janakiraman N, Nanda R, Uribe FA (2017) Targeted mechanics for treatment of patients with severe short-root anomaly. J Clin Orthod 51(5):279–289
92. Galhotra V, Pandit IK, Srivastava N, Gugnani N (2007) Endodontic treatment of a multirooted permanent maxillary canine. J Dent Child (Chic) 74(1):73–75
93. Ahmed HM, Hashem AA (2016) Accessory roots and root canals in human anterior teeth: a review and clinical considerations. Int Endod J 49(8):724–736
94. Rana V, Shafi S, Gambhir N, Rehani U (2011) Deciduous mandibular second molar with supernumerary roots and root canals associated with missing mandibular permanent premolar. Int J Clin Pediatr Dent 4(2):167–169
95. Kavanagh C, O'Sullivan VR (1998) A four-rooted primary upper second molar. Int J Paediatr Dent 8(4):279–282
96. Mochizuki K, Ohtawa Y, Kubo S, Machida Y, Yakushiji M (2001) Bifurcation, birooted primary canines: a case report. Int J Paediatr Dent 11(5):380–385
97. Song JS, Kim SO, Choi BJ, Choi HJ, Son HK, Lee JH (2009) Incidence and relationship of an additional root in the mandibular first permanent molar and primary molars. Oral Surg Oral Med Oral Pathol Oral Radiol Endod 107(1):e56–e60
98. Luder HU (2015) Malformations of the tooth root in humans. Front Physiol 6:307
99. Ahmed HM, Abbott PV (2012) Accessory roots in maxillary molar teeth: a review and endodontic considerations. Aust Dent J 57(2):123–31; quiz 248

Anomalies of Enamel Formation

7

7.1 Introduction

Enamel covers the crown of the tooth and is the most highly calcified substance in the body. It contains 96% mineralized substance with 4% organic materials [1]. The cells that are responsible for the formation of enamel are no longer present after tooth eruption and therefore, enamel is considered non-vital and unable to regenerate [1]. During amelogenesis, the enamel matrix is formed first followed by mineralization. The first layer of enamel formed is called the aprismatic layer. This layer lies next to dentin and forms the dentinoenamel junction (DEJ). After formation of this layer, the ameloblasts continue to form prismatic enamel as they retreat away from the aprismatic layer. The precise method of enamel mineralization is not quite understood; however, there are a few theories that describe a sequential process. One such theory describes how mineralization occurs in two stages. During the first stage, the enamel is mineralized 20–30% followed by the second stage where the enamel becomes fully mineralized. Another theory describes mineralization occurring in four stages. The first stage involves a very heavy mineralization of the aprismatic enamel layer located at the DEJ. This is followed by a 20–30% mineralization of all of the enamel, starting at the enamel surface and moving toward the DEJ. The next stage involves complete mineralization of all of the enamel but moving in an opposite direction to the prior stage (DEJ to enamel surface). During the final stage, the outermost enamel (few micrometers at the enamel surface) becomes highly calcified [1]. Enamel anomalies have multiple etiologies (genetic, systemic, local, or unknown causes), and can result in various clinical presentations depending on the cause and the stage of enamel formation.

J. A. Soxman et al., *Anomalies of the Developing Dentition*,
https://doi.org/10.1007/978-3-030-03164-0_7

7.2 Hereditary Amelogenesis Imperfecta

7.2.1 Description

Amelogenesis imperfecta (AI) is a hereditary condition affecting both the primary and permanent dentitions that results in abnormal quantitative/qualitative enamel formation [2]. As a hereditary condition, it is unrelated to various syndromic conditions that may have defective enamel as part of the systemic disease. AI affects an estimated one in 14,000 in the USA [3] and has been classified into four categories with multiple subtypes based on the mode of inheritance and phenotypic presentation [4, 5]. The hypoplastic type is the most frequent form of AI (61.2%) followed by hypomaturation AI (32.2%) and then by both the hypocalcified AI and mixed hypomaturation/hypoplastic AI (3.2%) [6].

Three major structural proteins are involved:

- Amelogenin is the most abundant [7].
- Amelobastin comprises approximately 5% of enamel protein [7].
- Enamelin is the largest protein but is least abundant [7].

Four genes (below) and 24 mutations are involved with AI in humans [7–9]:

- ENAM (enamelin gene)
- AMELX/AMELY (amelogenin gene on X/Y chromosome)
- MMP20 (matrix metalloproteinase 20/enamelysin gene)
- KLK4 (kallikrein 4 gene)

Patients affected by AI have increased sensitivity to hot and cold, and they have a reduced esthetic appearance due to discoloration of the anterior teeth and experience a decrease in masticatory function. Due to loss of enamel, there is a lack of interproximal contacts and a loss of vertical dimension [6].

As a result of the condition, patients affected by AI also experience psychosocial difficulties as they relate to social interaction anxiety measures, self-image and self-esteem measures, and self-perceived quality-of-life measures [10].

7.2.2 Etiology (Four Types of AI)

Type I, Hypoplastic AI is the most common form of AI. Since disruption occurs during the secretory stage of enamel formation, the enamel does not reach normal thickness [2, 7]. The subtypes of Hypoplastic AI (Table 7.1) describe the teeth as having different surface textures caused by defects in enamel formation to include enamel agenesis [6]. Although defective in amount, calcification does occur resulting in hard enamel [11]. Radiographically, the enamel has normal radiodensity while the thickness is markedly reduced [6].

Table 7.1 Molecular and physical properties of AI Type I (Hypoplastic AI)[a]

Hypoplastic AI Type I	Mode of inheritance	Enamel features Locally/generally thin enamel	Gene type
Subtype IA	Autosomal dominant	Small pits in rows/columns w/brown discolored bottom	ENAM
Subtype IB	Autosomal dominant	Horizontal pits/grooves in mid-third of crowns	ENAM
Subtype IC	Autosomal recessive	Like IB but more severe w/local hypocalcifications	ENAM
Subtype ID	Autosomal dominant	Smooth, glossy, no proximal contacts, white–brown, 50% anterior open-bite	ENAM
Subtype IE	X-linked males (10% of males)	Smooth, shiny, no proximal contacts, yellow–brown, anterior open-bite	AMELY
Subtype IE	X-linked females	Alternating thin/normal vertical bands (lyonization), 33% open-bite	AMELX
Subtype IF	Autosomal dominant	Rough, granular, glassy, no proximal contacts, 50% anterior open-bite	ENAM
Subtype IG	Autosomal recessive	Rough, granular, thin/absent, yellow–brown crowns, anterior open-bite	ENAM

[a]Table adapted from text: Pathology of Hard Dental Tissues (2013)

Table 7.2 Molecular and physical properties of AI Type II (hypomaturation AI)[a]

Hypomaturation AI Type II	Mode of inheritance	Enamel features Mottled, softer, normal thickness	Gene type
Subtype IIA	Autosomal recessive	Brownish, soft, chips away, normal thickness, anterior open-bite	MMP20 KLK4
Subtype IIB	X-linked males	Primary teeth are ground-glass white Permanent teeth are mottled yellow, thin, and smooth	AMELX
Subtype IIB	X-linked females	Primary teeth have vertical white/normal bands Permanent teeth have vertical white–yellow bands, soft	AMELX
Subtype IIC	X-linked	Snow-capped teeth[b]	AMELX
Subtype IID	Autosomal dominant	Snow-capped teeth[b]	

[a]Table adapted from text: Pathology of Hard Dental Tissues (2013)
[b]Snow-capped teeth is described as 1/4 to 1/3 of the incisal/occlusal part of the tooth having an opaque white color and porous

Type II, Hypomaturation AI is due to the failure in removal of the organic matrix and failure to promote the hardening of the enamel layer resulting in soft enamel [7]. As mentioned earlier, the phenotypic presentation varies depending on the genotype (Table 7.2). For example, the autosomal recessive form results in enamel that is mottled brown–yellow–white, is of normal thickness, soft, and tends to chip. The X-linked women carriers may have vertical lines of opaque white enamel alternating with bands of normal enamel (Lyon effect) [12]. In some types of hypomaturation AI, the defects in mineralization are mainly limited to the incisal or occlusal enamel of the anterior and posterior teeth, respectively, resulting in a snow-capped appearance [2]. Radiographically, there is decreased radiodensity.

Table 7.3 Molecular and physical properties of AI Type III (hypocalcified AI)[a]

Hypocalcified AI Type III	Mode of inheritance	Enamel features Very soft, normal thickness	Gene type
Subtype IIIA	Autosomal dominant	Yellow–brown/orange to brown–black (color change due to food staining)	Unknown
Subtype IIIB	Autosomal recessive	Similar to IIIA but more severe	Unknown

[a]Table adapted from text: Pathology of Hard Dental Tissues (2013)

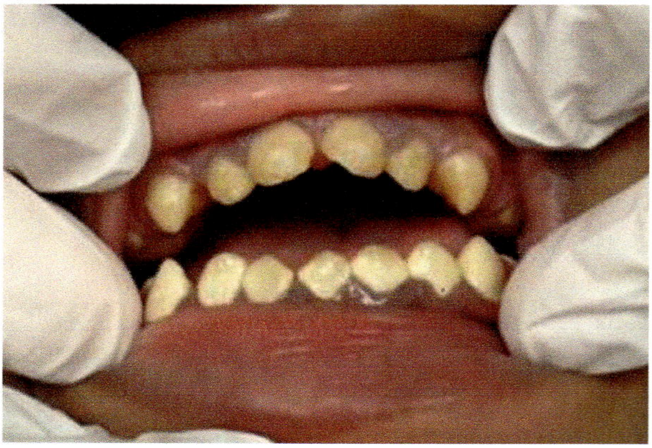

Fig. 7.1 Photograph of a patient with amelogenesis imperfecta and heavy calculus formation in the mandibular anterior teeth. (Courtesy of Dr. Tiffany Williams)

Type III, Hypocalcified AI initially develops normal thickness but consists of poorly calcified matrix, which is rapidly lost leaving exposed dentin (Table 7.3). Newly erupted teeth are yellow–orange in appearance and later can become more brown–black in appearance due to foods staining the poorly calcified enamel. Patients with hypocalcifed enamel develop calculus quickly (Fig. 7.1), since the enamel surface is rough [7]. Radiographically, enamel is less radiopaque than dentin.

Type IV, Hypomaturative-hypoplastic with taurodontism AI (AIHHT) presents with enamel that is mottled white–yellow–brown with pits most frequently on the labial surface (Fig. 7.2) or is thin with areas of hypomaturation (Table 7.4). Molar teeth can have taurodontic pulp chambers [13], while other teeth may have enlarged pulp chambers. AIHHT is a distinct entity in that it is one of the phenotypes present in patients diagnosed with tricho–dento–osseous syndrome (TDO). TDO is due to a DLX3 mutation and primarily affects hair, teeth, and bones; therefore, the syndrome consists of kinky hair, dysplastic nails, sclerotic bones, enamel hypoplasia, and severe taurodontism [9]. For patients who present with the AIHHT without the hair and boney defects, the molecular defect for AIHHT alone remains to be discovered [14]. Radiographically, the enamel has approximately the same or greater radiodensity than dentin [5].

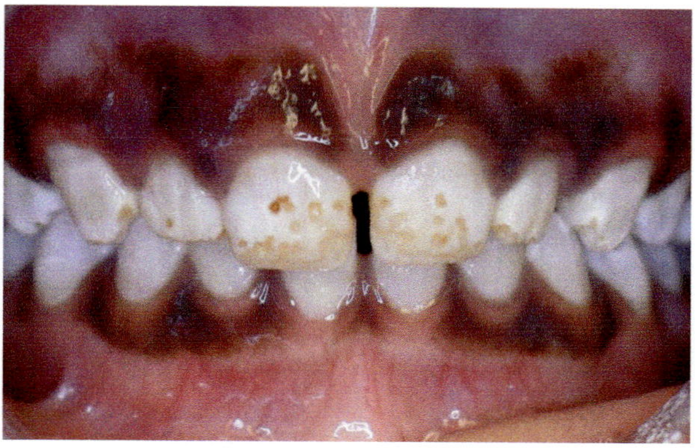

Fig. 7.2 Photograph of a patient with amelogenesis imperfecta showing pitting of the enamel surface. (Courtesy of Dr. Reham AlNajjar)

Table 7.4 Molecular and physical properties of AI Type IV (AIHHT)[a]

AIHHT Type IV	Mode of inheritance	Enamel features Localized thin areas, mottled, soft, radiodensity similar to that of dentin	Gene type
Subtype IVA	Autosomal dominant	Soft, mottled yellow–brown and opaque white, with pits	Unknown
Subtype IVB	Autosomal dominant	Thin and soft with hypomaturative areas	Unknown

[a]Table adapted from text: Pathology of Hard Dental Tissues (2013)

7.2.3 Treatment/Management

There is a decreased longevity of restorations in patients with AI. The survival rate after 5 years is only 50% with the survivability being relative to the severity of the condition. The various types of AI resulted in different survival rates with higher survival rates occurring with the hypoplastic type than with the hypomaturation or hypocalcification types [6].

When considering restorative treatment for AI patients, one must keep in mind that optimal patient management takes into consideration the phase of dental development. Treating patients in the mixed dentition can be complex and there is currently no standard of care established for managing the AI-affected patient during the mixed dentition stage [15]. Preservation of tooth structure should be the goal, and treatment provided for permanent teeth should be conservative in the mixed dentition when considering the fact that over-prepared molars and incisors will be difficult to restore with more definitive cast crowns later. Studies have recommended restorative materials such as glass ionomer, resins, amalgam, and stainless steel crowns (Fig. 7.3). The authors have reported failure of resin restorations on teeth with AI and when provided, they recommend that resin restorations should be considered interim restorations until more definite restorative care could be provided; however, patients did experience relief from sensitivity and better self-esteem because of the early restorative care [6, 15].

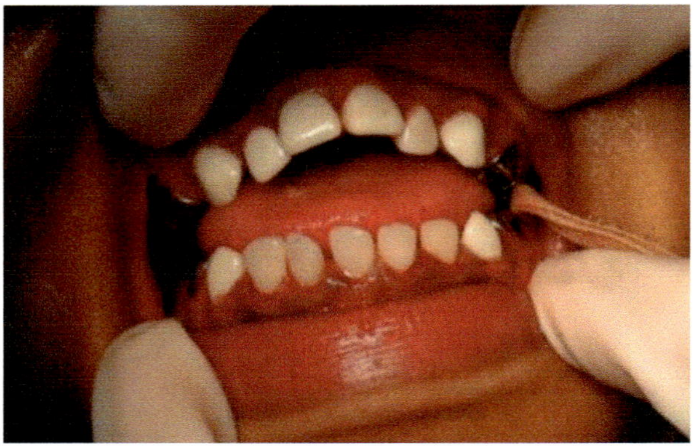

Fig. 7.3 Photograph following a full mouth dental rehabilitation in the operating room with anterior zirconia crowns used to restore the anterior teeth and stainless steel crowns used to restore the posterior teeth. (Courtesy of Dr. Tiffany Williams)

Hypomineralization is more severe with the hypocalcifed and hypomaturation types of AI. Restoration of hypomineralized enamel may be more successful by pretreating the enamel with 5% sodium hypochlorite to remove protein that has encased hydroxyapatite [16].

7.3 Molar Incisor Hypomineralization (MIH)

7.3.1 Description

MIH is an enamel developmental defect of unknown systemic origin of the first permanent molars (Fig. 7.4), frequently associated with similar defects of the incisor teeth with a prevalence rate of 2.8–25% [6] (Fig. 7.5).

7.3.2 Etiology

Although the cause may be unclear, there may be multifactorial factors that predispose patients to this condition such as children who are born preterm, those with poor general health, or systemic conditions that occur within their first 3 years of development [16]. MIH is characterized by demarcated opacities that vary from white to brown in color and due to a porous subsurface, the enamel is prone to post-eruptive breakdown [17]. Hypersensitivity is a frequent complaint most likely due to the constant pulpal inflammation that is present under the opaque area thereby making it difficult for local anesthetic effectiveness in pain control [17]. According to a study performed by Jose da Silva Figueiredo Se et al., there is an association between the prevalence of MIH in primary second molars and primary canines with the presence of MIH in the permanent dentition. The importance of these findings leaves the provider with the opportunity to recognize the condition early (in the primary dentition) in order to intervene with preventive measures as soon as the permanent teeth begin to erupt.

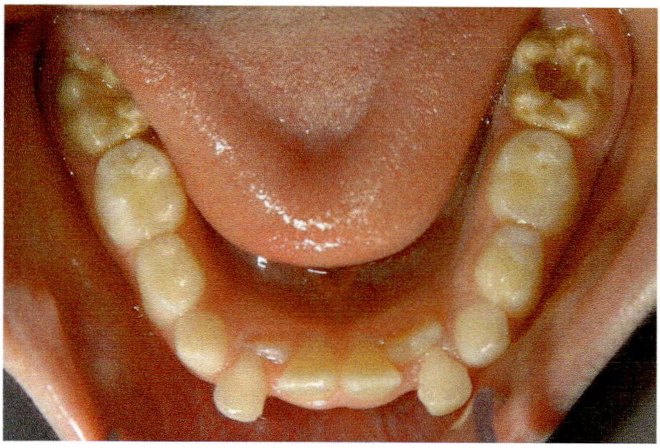

Fig. 7.4 Photograph showing hypomineralization of the permanent first mandibular molars

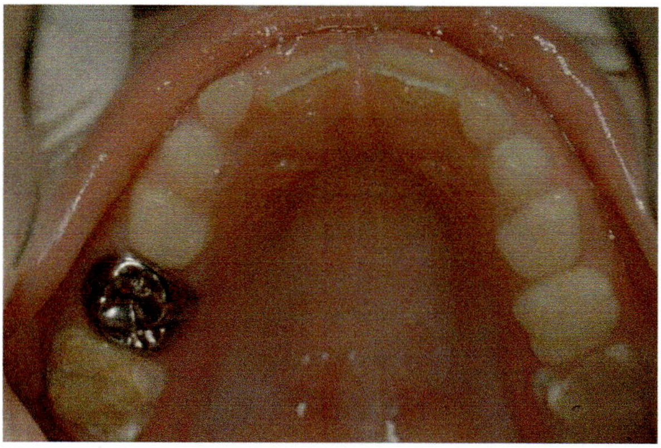

Fig. 7.5 Photograph showing hypomineralization of both the permanent central incisors and first permanent molars in a patient with molar incisor hypomineralization

7.3.3 Treatment/Management

Depending on the severity of destruction, treatment can be more preventive by employing remineralization/desensitizing strategies, restorative care ranging from sealants to full coverage restorations, and extractions for the more severely affected teeth. Restoring affected permanent first molars can be difficult due to ineffectiveness of local anesthesia, child behavior management, ensuring the adequate removal of the affected enamel, and selecting an appropriate restorative material [16]. It is recommended to treat as early as possible to halt the destructive effects on the dentition [18].

Preventive:

- Casein phospho-peptide-amorphous calcium phosphate (CPP-ACP)
  - Creates a state of supersaturation followed by deposition of calcium and phosphate ions at the enamel surface [16]

- Fluoride
  - Varnish and gels
- Desensitizing toothpaste

Restorative:

- Glass ionomers
  - Used for dentin replacement or as an interim restoration
  - Advantage of placement ease, fluoride release, and chemical bonding
  - Disadvantage is that they are not recommended for stress-bearing areas
  - Types
    Glass ionomer
    Resin-modified glass ionomer
- Resin composites
  - Useful for one- or two-surface well-demarcated enamel defects without cuspal involvement, margins must be on sound enamel
  - Advantages
    Good handling
    High wear resistance
    Adhesion achieved through the use of resin-based adhesives
  - Disadvantages
    Technique sensitivity (moisture control)
- Amalgams
  - Amalgam can be used similarly to composite in areas where moisture control is difficult
- Stainless Steel Crowns
  - Stainless steel crowns are indicated to restore more severely affected teeth where cusps are involved

7.4 Enamel Hypoplasia/Turner's Tooth

7.4.1 Description

Enamel hypoplasia resembling AI can be associated with a number of syndromes or as part of a medical condition. As mentioned previously, AIHHT is associated with TDO syndrome. Acquired systemic causes generally result in a more generalized presentation of the enamel defects, whereas the acquired local causes are more likely to result in affecting one or two teeth.

Enamel hypoplasia may be mild resulting in pitting of the enamel surface or be more severe resulting in the development of horizontal lines in the enamel across the crown surface (whereas genetic AI are vertical) (Fig. 7.6). It can occur in either the primary or permanent dentition or both, with the primary dentition generally being less severe and related to the complications of premature birth [11].

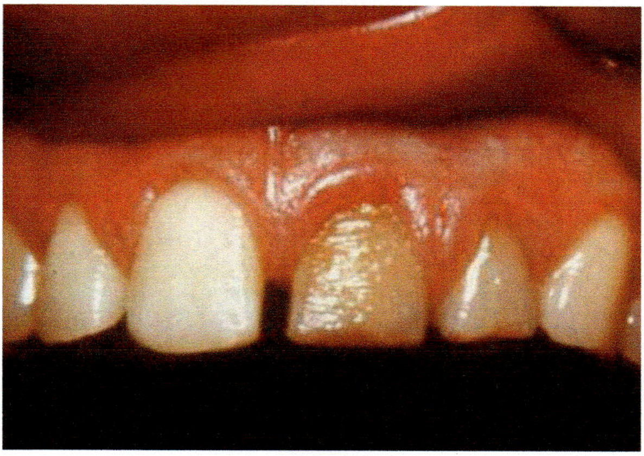

Fig. 7.6 Photograph of Turner's tooth; note the horizontal lines across the enamel surface of the left central incisor. (Courtesy of Dr. John Svirsky)

7.4.2 Etiology

Acquired systemic causes [11, 19]

- Environmental
  - Possible causes
    Nutritional (vitamins A, C, and D, calcium, phosphate, and magnesium)
    GI disorders (celiac disease) [20]
    Phenylketonuria
    Allergies (congenital allergies, not seasonal)
    Chronic fluorosis
    Drugs (Tetracycline)
    Lead poisoning (plumbism)
    Ionizing radiation and chemotherapy (for treatment of Acute Lymphoblastic Leukemia in children)
    Rubella embryopathy (anomalies due to in utero infection with Rubella)
    Presence of high fever at a young age [21]
- Chromosomal Defects and Syndromes
  - Nephrotic syndrome
  - Cleft Lip Cleft Palate
- Brain Injury and Neurologic Defects (Cerebral Palsy)

Acquired local causes

- Infection
  - Turner tooth is described as enamel hypoplasia occurring in a permanent tooth due to a local infection of a primary anterior or posterior tooth [11].
  - The retention of infected primary teeth that are asymptomatic is unacceptable [11].
- Trauma
  - Turner's hypoplasia of a permanent incisor can be a result of localized trauma of an anterior primary tooth, most likely intrusion or avulsion [22].

- Falls can result in a traumatic blow to an anterior primary tooth resulting in its displacement into the permanent developing successor. The trauma or subsequent infection produces defects on the labial surface on the permanent successor.
- The frequency of developmental disturbances found in a permanent tooth directly relates the severity of traumatic injury to its primary tooth predecessor [23]; however, factors such as age at the time of incident, degree of root resorption of the injured primary tooth, the type and extent of traumatic lesion, and the stage of development of the permanent tooth germ are factors that can have an effect on the severity [24].
- According to a study performed by Skarre et al.:

  The most common permanent tooth sequel to primary tooth trauma was discoloration of the permanent tooth.

  Hypoplasia was observed in 5% of the successors following trauma, whereas diffuse opacities were observed in 13% due to other causes.
- Laryngoscopy and endotracheal intubation can result in trauma to the primary incisors resulting in enamel defects of the permanent successor (primarily affects left maxillary incisors) [11].

7.4.3 Treatment/Management

Treatment of teeth with enamel hypoplasia is similar to that of AI and MIH.

Treatment will depend on the severity and extensiveness of the enamel defect, which can affect the effectiveness of the dental materials used to restore teeth [21]. Scheidt et al. studied the difference in shear bond strength between hypoplastic primary teeth as compared to primary teeth with healthy enamel and found that there was no significant difference. However, they found that there were more cohesive and mixed fractures in the hypoplastic group and therefore recommended roughening the hypoplastic enamel before etching and bonding to improve the bond strength of the final restoration [21].

7.5 Opaque Enamel Spots

7.5.1 Description

Terms used to describe opaque enamel spots include "flecks" in the enamel, "white spots" in the enamel, and "mottled enamel." However, a mottled defect appears posteruptively and then increases with pigmentation with age, especially in tooth surfaces exposed to light when the lips are parted [25]. Opaque enamel spots are developmental in origin and as the affected tooth erupts, they are visibly present (Fig. 7.7). They can occur in the anterior or posterior teeth with the former usually presenting with smaller lesions facially (Figs. 7.8 and 7.9) and the latter affecting one cusp or the entire crown of the tooth [25].

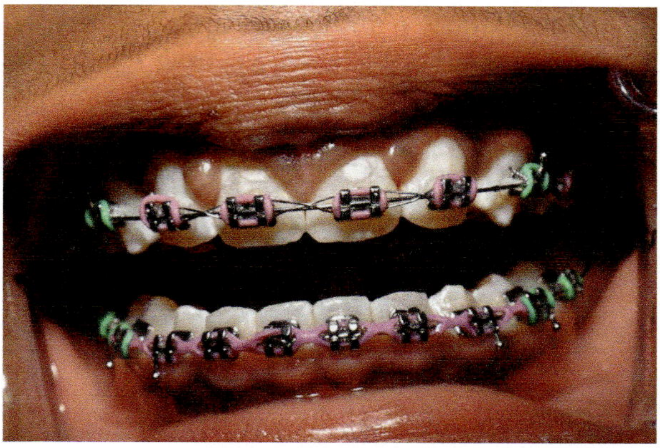

Fig. 7.7 Photograph of enamel opaque spots on the anterior teeth that were present prior to the initiation of orthodontic treatment. Note gingival location of the opaque white spots that were not apparent until the central permanent incisors were fully erupted

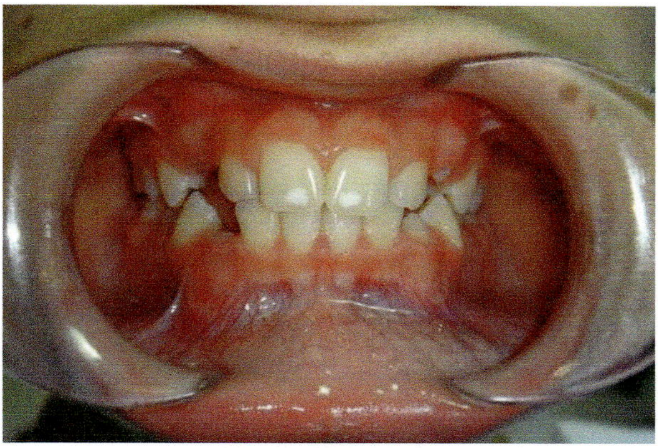

Fig. 7.8 Photograph of enamel white spots on the upper right and upper left permanent central incisors

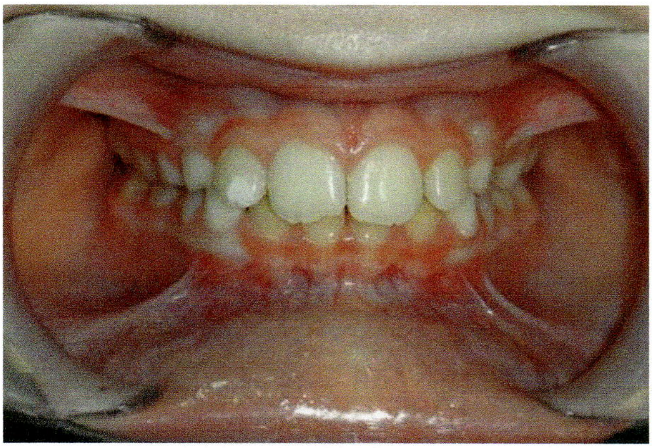

Fig. 7.9 Photograph of enamel white spot on the upper right permanent lateral incisor

7.5.2 Etiology

Opaque enamel spots are not due to dental fluorosis but may be attributed to possible systemic conditions [25]. Opaque white spots can occur after orthodontic treatment due to the entrapment of plaque around the orthodontic brackets; also, the appliances tend to shift the lesions from the posterior to anterior teeth and from interproximal to vestibular and lingual sites [26].

7.5.3 Treatment

The occurrence of enamel opaque spots or white spot lesions is high after orthodontic treatment (61%) and it is believed that natural salivary remineralization of these lesions can occur over time; however, there is little improvement of the esthetics or structural properties of the deeper lesions [27]. Developmental enamel opaque spots, depending on the size and location, will warrant treatment for esthetic or functional concerns.

- Remineralization
  - Casein phosphopeptides work by increasing the levels of calcium and phosphate ions in the subsurface of lesion resulting in subsurface remineralization and a more esthetic outcome [27].
  - Concentrated fluoride in not recommended for the treatment of these lesions since it will result in hypermineralization, which in effect maintains the whiteness of these lesions.
- Restoration [28]
  - Conservative treatment of enamel opaque spots or white spot lesions can be performed through the use of superficial or deep infiltration of composite resin.

    A 15% hydrochloric acid solution is used to access the hypomineralized lesion.

    An extremely fluid resin is infiltrated into the body of the lesion (Icon: DMG, Hamburg Germany).

    Resin infiltration into demineralized enamel increases the mechanical resistance and also improves the translucency of the enamel surface thereby improving the strength and esthetics of the treated surface.

References

1. Gartner LP (1999) Dentin. Essential of oral histology and embryology, Chap. 3, 3rd edn. Jen House, Baltimore, pp 31, 45, 52
2. Backman B, Holm AK (1986) Amelogenesis imperfecta: prevalence and incidence in a northern Swedish county. Community Dent Oral Epidemiol 14:43–47
3. Collins MA, Mauriello SM, Tyndall DA, Wright JT (1999) Dental anomalies associated with amelogenesis imperfecta. Oral Surg Oral Med Oral Pathol Oral Radiol Endod 88:358–364

4. Aldred MJ, Savarirayan R, Crawford PJW (2003) Amelogenesis imperfecta: a classification and catalogue for the 21st century. Oral Dis 9:19–23
5. Witkop CJ Jr (1989) Amelogenesis imperfecta, dentinogenesis imperfecta and dentin dysplasia revisited: problems in classification. J Oral Pathol 17:547–553
6. Sabandal MMI, Schafer E (2016) Amelogenesis imperfecta: review of diagnostic findings and treatment concepts. Odontology 104:245–256
7. Hu JC, Chun YH, Hazzazzi T, Simmer JP (2007) Enamel formation and amelogenesis imperfecta. Cells Tissues Organs 186:78–85
8. Ozdemir D, Hart PS, Ryu OH, Choi SJ, Ozdemir-Karatas M, Firatli E, Piesco N, Hart TC (2005) MMP20 active-site mutation in hypomaturation amelogenesis imperfecta. J Dent Res 84(11):1031–1035
9. Seow WK (1993) Clinical diagnosis and management strategies of amelogenesis imperfecta variants. Pediatr Dent 15(6):384–393
10. Coffield KD, Hillips C, Brady M, Roberts MW, Strauss RP, Wright T (2005) The psychosocial impact of developmental dental defects in people with hereditary amelogenesis imperfecta. J Am Dent Assoc 136:620–630
11. Dean JA (2016) McDonald and Avery's dentistry for the child and adolescent, 10th edn. Elsevier, St. Louis, pp 51, 59–61
12. Lench NJ, Winter GB (1995) Characterization of molecular defects in X-linked amelogenesis imperfecta (A1H1). Hum Mutat 5:251–259
13. Klein U, Paimagham B, Blumhagen R, Kroehl M, Sain J (2017) Pyramidal and taurodont molars and their association with other tooth anomalies. Pediatr Dent 39(1):46–52
14. Wright TJ (2006) The molecular etiologies and associated phenotypes of amelogenesis imperfecta. Am J Med Genet 140A:2547–2555
15. Chen CF, Hu JCC, Padilla Estrella MR, Peters MC, Bresciani E (2013) Assessment of restorative treatment of patients with amelogenesis imperfecta. Pediatr Dent 35(4):337–342
16. William V, Messer LB, Burrow MF (2006) Molar incisor hypomineralization review and recommendations for clinical management. Pediatr Dent 28(3):224–232
17. Da Silva Figueiredo Se MJ, Dias Ribeiro AP, Martins dos Santos-Pinto LA, Loiola Cordeiro RC, Cabral RN, Leal SC (2017) Are hypomineralized primary molars and canines associated with molar-incisor hypominerlization? Pediatr Dent 39(7):445–449
18. Segun A, Ozer F (2002) Restoring function and esthetics in a patient with amelogenesis imperfecta: a case report. Quintessence Int 33(3):199–204
19. El-Najjar MY, Desante MV, Ozebek L (1978) Prevalence and possible etiology of dental enamel hypoplasia. Am J Phys Anthropol 48:185–192
20. Ferraz EG, Campos Ede J, Sarmento VA, Silva LR (2012) The oral manifestations of celiac disease: information for the pediatric dentist. Pediatr Dent 34(7):485–488
21. Scheidt L, Sanabe ME, Collares FM, Leitune VCB, Bresciani E, Diniz MB (2016) Assessment of enamel bond strength of hypoplastic primary teeth. Pediatr Dent 38(5):432–436
22. Bhushan BA, Garg S, Sharma D, Jain M (2008) Esthetic and endosurgical management of Turner's hypoplasia; a sequlae of trauma to developing tooth germ. J Indian Soc Pedod Prev Dent 26:121–124
23. Skarre AB, Maseng AL, Wand NJ (2015) Enamel defects on permanent successors following luxation injuries to primary teeth and carers' experiences. Int J Paediatr Dent 25:221–228
24. de Amorim Lde F, Estrela C, da Costa LR (2011) Effects of traumatic dental injuries to primary teeth on permanent teeth—a clinical follow-up study. Dent Traumatol 27:117–121
25. Hurme VO (1949) Developmental opacities of teeth in a New England community. Am J Dis Child 77(1):61–75
26. Mizrahi E (1983) Surface distribution of enamel opacities following orthodontic treatment. Am J Orthod 84(4):323–331
27. Chen H, Liu X, Dai J, Jiang Z, Guo T, Ding Y (2013) Effect of remineralizing agents on white spot lesions after orthodontic treatment: a systematic review. Am J Orthod Dentofac Orthop 143(3):376–382
28. Attal JP, Atlan A, Denis M, Vennat E, Tirlet G (2014) White spots on enamel: treatment protocol by superficial or deep infiltration (part 2). Int Orthod 12:1–31

8 Anomalies of Dentin Formation

8.1 Introduction

Dentin forms the major hard tissue component of the tooth and unlike enamel and cementum, it is present in both the crown and root of the tooth. It is highly elastic and therefore performs efficiently under the highly calcified and brittle enamel. It is considered to be a living tissue since in contains long odontoblastic processes within its dentinal tubules which originate in the pulp [1]. Dentin by weight is composed of approximately 70% inorganic mineral, 20% organic matrix, and 10% water. The organic matrix consists primarily of type I collagen (about 85%) followed by acidic proteins and proteoglycans [2]. According to Sauk et al., Type I collagen is the only known type of collagen molecule of normal mature bone and dentin [3]. The result of normal dentin formation is the presence of dentinal tubules that run throughout the dentin layer from the mantle layer of dentin to the inner layer of circumpulpal dentin without interruption. The outermost layer of the dentin consists of mantle dentin, which is the first layer of dentin formed followed by the primary dentin layer (circumpulpal dentin) that makes up the bulk of the dentin. The formation of primary dentin occurs prior to the completion of root formation and secondary dentin occurs subsequent to root completion but not in the response to trauma as tertiary dentin is [1] (Fig. 8.1).

Dentinogenesis is a strictly controlled process that results in the conversion of unmineralized predentin to mineralized dentin [2]. Anomalies that affect the formation of dentin are primarily genetic. One must understand normal dentin formation to understand the differences between the various dentinal defects. In general, defects in dentin formation occur during the histodifferentiation, when cells of the dental papilla differentiate to become preodontoblasts that eventually elaborate to become the dental matrix, or during apposition, when the preodontoblasts begin to elaborate the dentin matrix, composed of Type I collagen, and become odontoblasts [4]. Defects during histodifferentiation result in a condition called dentinogenesis imperfecta and defects during apposition result in dentinal dysplasia, with both

J. A. Soxman et al., *Anomalies of the Developing Dentition*,
https://doi.org/10.1007/978-3-030-03164-0_8

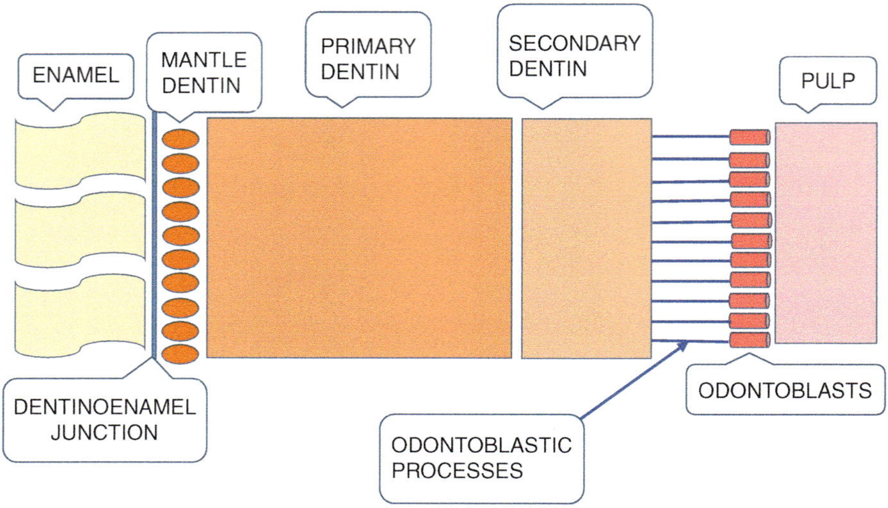

Fig. 8.1 Diagram of dentin

resulting from abnormalities in the dental papilla, the mesenchymal part of the tooth germ, that results in the formation of dysfunctional odontoblasts [2]. A major component of the noncollagenous dentin matrix of normal human dentin is a highly phosphorylated protein called dentin phosphophoryn (DP). This protein is limited to the circumpulpal dentin and is not present in mantle, reparative, or secondary dentins; therefore, DP is secreted by fully differentiated odontoblasts and not from those that are undifferentiated or degenerated [5]. In a study by Takgi et al., the authors discuss how the causative factors for DI Types I and II may be due to undifferentiated or degenerated "scleroblasts" which do not secrete phosphophoryn, as seen with mantel and reparative dentins. The authors continue to discuss how both DI Types I and II share a primary lesion of dentin formation due to a severely reduced life span of its odontoblast as compared to the long life span of the odontoblast in normal dentin [5].

Recent studies have found that defects in the dentin sialophosphoprotein (DSPP) gene cause DI Type II, DI Type III, and Dentinal Dysplasia Type II (DD Type II) [2, 6, 7]. Coster et al. describe DI Type I as a syndromic (osteogenesis imperfecta) heritable defective dentin condition and DI Types II and III as well as DD Type II as non-syndromic heritable defective dentin conditions where these latter conditions have no other gene mutation other than the DSPP gene [2].

In 1973, Shields et al. developed a classification of hereditary dentin defects and discovered that the one unifying factor was that the condition affected both primary and permanent dentitions, and that there was a common time for the initiation of the defect since all affected teeth have normal mantle dentin. Shields also developed two broad identifiable categories, dentinogenesis imperfecta with three subcategories and dentin dysplasia with two subcategories [8] (Table 8.1).

Table 8.1 Differential diagnosis of dentinal defects

	DD-I	DD-II	DI-I	DI-II	DI-III
Clinical					
1. Primary teeth amber/translucent	N	Y	V	Y	V
2. Permanent teeth discolored	N	N	N	Y	N
3. Discoloration in both dentitions	N	N	Y	Y	Y
4. Rapid attrition of crowns	N	N	V	Y	Y
Radiographic					
1. Short, tapering roots	Y	N	V	V	V
2.a. Obliteration of the pulp before eruption	Y	N	V	V	V
2.b. Obliteration of the pulp after eruption	N	V	V	Y	V
3. Multiple apical radiolucencies	Y	N	V	V	V
4. Thistle-tube shape to the pulp chamber	N	V	N	N	N
5. Reduced radiographic contrast of the dentin	Y	N	Y	Y	V
6. Pulp stones in the pulp chamber	N	Y	N	N	N
Common features					
1. Primary teeth more severely affected	Y	Y	Y	Y	Y
2. Normal mantle dentin	Y	Y	Y	Y	Y
3. Abnormal radicular dentin	V	Y	Y	Y	Y
4. Normal enamel	Y	Y	V	V	V

Table adapted by Shields 1973
N absent or unreported, *V* variable in frequency or severity, *Y* typically evident in all teeth

8.2 Dentinogenesis Imperfecta

8.2.1 Description

Dentinogenesis imperfecta (DI) is a hereditary condition affecting both the primary and permanent dentitions that results in abnormal dentin formation and affects an estimated one in 8000 individuals [8, 9]. Earlier studies on DI referred to it as hereditary opalescent dentin due to the violet color of the enamel and the light to dark brown staining of exposed dentin [10]. Others have described it as teeth with a bluish brown color and normal enamel surface, an over-production of dentin resulting in complete obliteration of the pulp and atypical dentin displaying an increased dentin matrix with an irregular arrangement of dentinal tubules [11, 12]. Some studies have described the dentin as being soft leading to excessive wear and that the dentin contained an abundance of interglobular dentin with high moisture and low inorganic content [13]. In 1939, Hodge et al. summarized the clinical presentation of hereditary opalescent dentin as teeth of amber color and increased translucency and tendency to fracture/wear easily with a radiographic presentation of decreased root size, absence of pulp chambers, and partial/total obliteration of the pulp [14]. Clinically, in addition to the amber translucent color, the crowns of the teeth appear bulbous due to a constriction of the cervical portion of the root and the tapered and short "spike-like" root features [11].

8.3 Classification of Dentinogenesis Imperfecta

8.3.1 Description and Etiology of Each Subtype

Dentinogenesis Type I (Dentinogenesis Imperfecta/Osteogenesis Imperfecta)

- Clinical features
  - Amber translucency of the teeth (Fig. 8.2) occurs in both dentitions.
  - Enamel fracture away resulting in rapid wear of the underlying soft dentin (Figs. 8.3 and 8.4).
- Radiographic features
  - Pulpal obliteration occurs prior to or soon after eruption [8, 9].
  - The deciduous and early permanent teeth are affected by an accelerated obliteration of the pulp, therefore these teeth are the most severely affected [8].
- Pathologic features
  - The normal mantle dentin merges with a dysplastic form of dentin that eventually proliferates and obliterates the pulp [8].

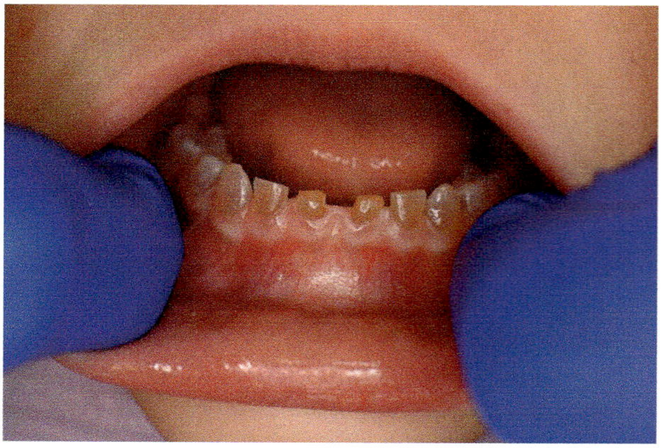

Fig. 8.2 Photograph showing the amber translucent appearance of the teeth

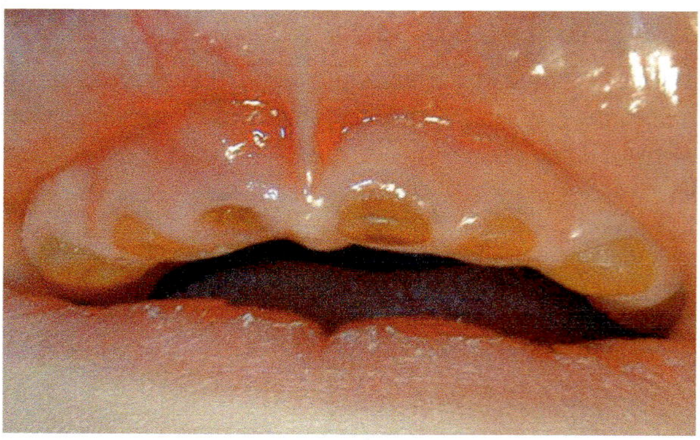

Fig. 8.3 Photograph showing the rapid wear of the dentin in the primary dentition

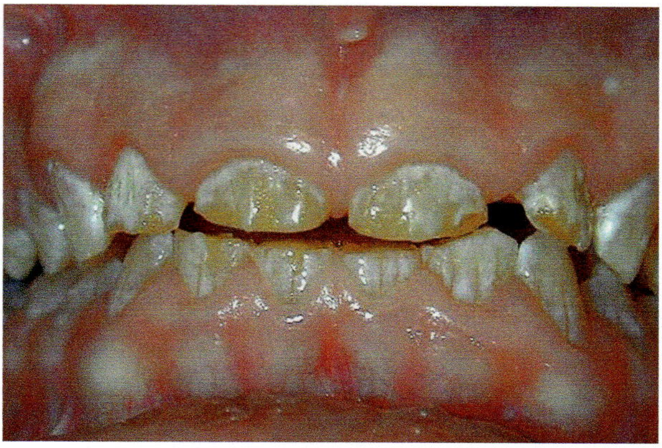

Fig. 8.4 Photograph showing how the enamel has fractured off with the resultant excessive wear of the underlying dentin in the permanent dentition

- Dentin is mostly atubular but if tubules exist, they show considerable variation in size and direction [8].
- True denticles occur within the affected dentin [8].

- Genetic considerations
  - DI-1 is the dental phenotype of patients affected with osteogenesis imperfecta (OI) [9, 15].

    OI is usually caused by defects in the two genes encoding type I collagen:

    COLIA1

    COLIA2
  - Degree of expressivity is variable, even within a single individual [9].

    Defects range from total pulpal obliteration to teeth with normal dentin and vascular canals [8].
- Other considerations [9]
  - DI Type I occurs in syndromes other than OI:

    Ehlers–Danlos syndrome

    Goldblatt syndrome

    Schimke immune-osseous dysplasia
  - DI Type I and DD phenotypes are becoming recognized as variable features in many syndromes [2].

Dentinogenesis Type II (Hereditary Opalescent Dentin)

- Most common type of DI [16]
- DI Type II has many clinical, radiographic, pathologic, and hereditary similarities to DI type I; the following features make it unique thus owing to its own classification:
  - Families with DI Type II have never had OI [8].
  - Within families, the severity of coloration and attrition is high for DI type II whereas with DI Type I the severity is more variable [8].
  - With DI Type II, both dentitions are equally affected both clinically and radiographically; one never finds completely normal teeth (whereas in DI Type I,

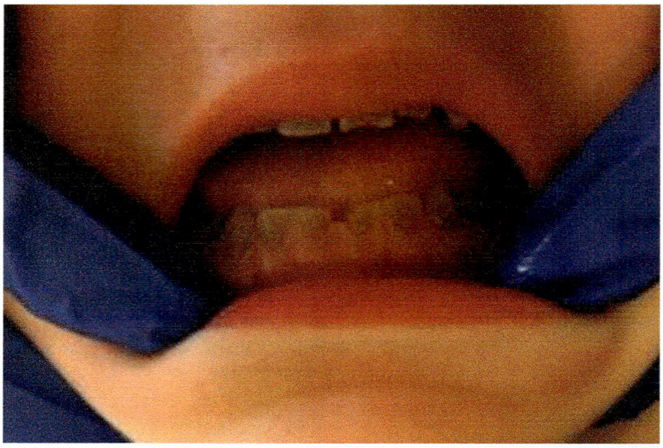

Fig. 8.5 Photograph of dentinogenesis imperfecta in the primary dentition. For DI Type I, the primary dentition is more severely affected than the permanent dentition. (Courtesy of Dr. Gail Kim)

the primary dentition is more severely affected (Fig. 8.5) than the permanent dentition and within the permanent dentition, it is not uncommon to find normal-appearing teeth) [17].

- Genetic considerations
  - Defects in the DSPP gene can cause DI Type II [9].
    "The gene product is a precursor protein that is cleaved into two dentin-specific matrix proteins" [18]:
    Dentin sialoprotein (DSP)
    Dentin phosphoprotein (DPP)

Dentinogenesis Type III (Brandywine Isolate Hereditary Opalescent Dentin)

- Description
  - Extremely rare condition found in a triracial isolate from Brandywine, MD [16].
    Triracial isolate in the USA consists of Native American Indians, African Americans, and Caucasians of European decent [7].
- Clinical features
  - Characterized by multiple pulpal exposures in the primary dentition [8].
  - Affected teeth vary in color and shape [8].
- Radiographic features
  - Vary in appearance from having:
    Normal dentin [8]
    Dentin similar in appearance to dentin of DI Type II [8]
    Teeth have a hollow appearance "shell" teeth (condition where after the mantle layer of dentin is formed, dentin formation stops leaving only the mantle layer that appears shell-like) [8]; according to Kim and Simmer, this is not unique to DI Type III since the pulp of DI Type II teeth are initially wide and appear shell-like but do obliterate over time [9]
    Some teeth have spherical bodies within the pulp (denticles) similar to DD Type I [19]

- Genetic considerations
  - Autosomal dominant [8]
  - There is a similar genotype between DI Type II and III since the DSPP mutation has been discovered in different families with varying phenotypic presentations of either DI Type II or III [9, 17]

8.3.2 Treatment

The dentist plays an important role in treating patients with DI. Early diagnosis and treatment are imperative to contribute to an improved quality of life for the patient. The progression of caries is slow due to rapid attrition of the teeth attributable to the soft underlying dentin [16]. The weakened state of the teeth warrants early treatment that can help eliminate many problems such as a loss in vertical dimension and interproximal space due to the breakdown caused by rapid occlusal attrition or due to extractions of nonrestorable-affected teeth [15]. Early treatment can also aid in preventing the psychological aspects related to patients who have discolored teeth and malocclusion [15].

Treatment can vary depending on the age of the patient and severity of the condition; therefore, treatment plans are highly individualized and should begin as early as possible, in the primary dentition, and managed throughout the mixed into the permanent dentition stage of development [15, 17].

Dental therapies should take in consideration normal dental development, vertical dimension, and esthetics [15].

Treatment is multidisciplinary and can include [16]:

- Full coverage restorations
  - Primary teeth

    Stainless steel crowns for the primary molar teeth

    Composite strip, stainless steel with white facing or ceramic crowns for the primary anterior teeth
  - Permanent teeth full cast or ceramic crowns

    Mixed dentition stainless steel crowns for the permanent first and second molars

    Permanent dentition full cast crowns after the pubertal growth spurt
- Over dentures or partial dentures maintain intra- and inter-arch relationships
- Orthognathic surgery to correct severe malocclusions
- Orthodontics to correct alignment of the teeth for better function and esthetics

The endodontic implications surrounding the treatment of teeth with DI include [11]:

- Determine pulp vitality
  - Cold test

    Patients with DI will respond to cold tests since the dentinal tubules are larger in diameter and contain up to 60% more water than that of normal dentin thus prompting teeth to respond to cold more readily.
  - Electric pulp testing is not reliable due to the degree of pulpal calcification

- Prognosis poor due to the highly irregular and poorly mineralized dentin
- Elective endodontics recommended if necessary to assist in restoration of the teeth (post-space)

8.4 Dentinal Dysplasia

8.4.1 Description

Dentinal dysplasia (DD) is an extremely rare inherited dentin structural anomaly with no systemic background, and presents itself in both dentitions [19]. There is no predilection for either sex and there is a common time for initiation since all teeth have normal mantle dentin [8, 19]. Shields developed two subtypes based on clinical/radiographic appearance. DD Type I (radicular dentinal dysplasia) presents with normal crowns and short roots with pulpal obliteration. DD Type II (coronal dentinal dysplasia) features short boubous crowns that are yellow–brown in color with pulp obliteration in the primary dentition and in the permanent dentition, normal colored/shaped crowns with large pulp chambers that later obliterate with having near normal root structure [2].

DD Type I (radicular dentinal dysplasia) [2, 19]

- Affects only the radicular dentin of both the primary and permanent dentitions [2]
- Clinically, both the primary and permanent clinical crowns are usually normal in shape, form, and consistency [8], although they may appear slightly opalescent, bluish, or brownish [6]
- Clinically, normal attrition in both dentitions as compared to DI [2]
- Radiographically
  - The roots are short, sharp, conic, or absent ("rootless teeth") in both dentitions, resulting in mobility and early loss/exfoliation of the teeth [2, 19, 20]
  - Primary teeth present with obliterated pulp chambers (Fig. 8.6) and permanent teeth have crescent-shaped pulp chambers [20]. There are usually a

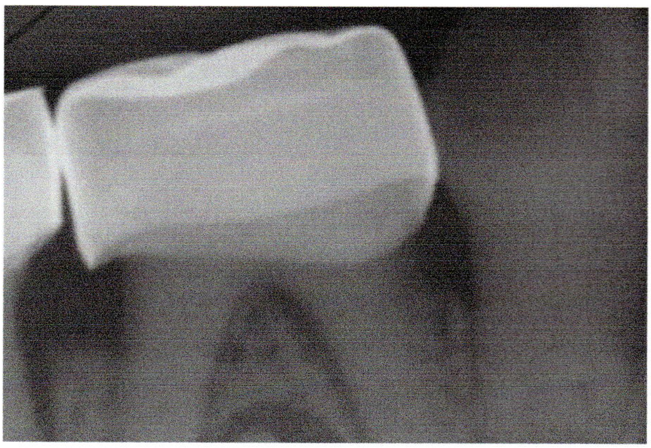

Fig. 8.6 Radiograph displaying the primary teeth with obliterated pulp chambers and canals

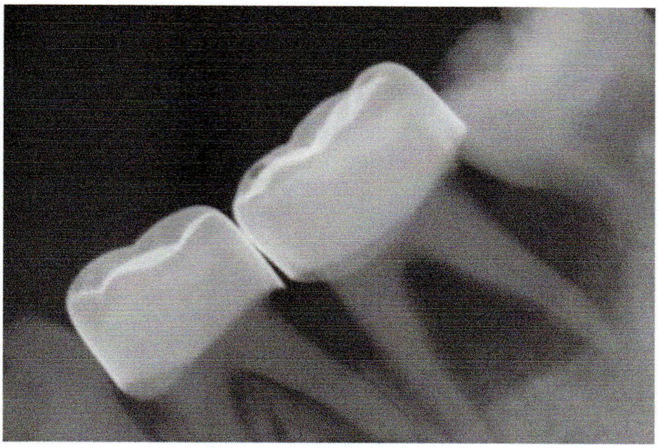

Fig. 8.7 Dentinal dysplasia type I with obliterated pulp and periradicular defect. (Courtesy of Dr. William Dahlke)

number of periapical radiolucencies (granulomas, cysts, or abscesses) in non-carious teeth which is pathognomonic for the condition [2, 8, 19, 20] (Fig. 8.7)
– Molars frequently present with severe taurodontism due to root fusion [6]

DD Type II (coronal dentinal dysplasia)

- Primary teeth have a similar clinical appearance to those with DI Type II (opalescent color) [2].
- Permanent teeth are normal in clinical appearance or have crowns that have a brown–gray discoloration [8].
- Radiographically, the roots of the permanent teeth are of normal length without evidence of periapical pathology; however, the pulp cavities may show a thistle-tube deformity and contain pulp stones. There have been reported cases of primary teeth having the same thistle-tube pulp chambers and pulp stones, and theorized that this presentation is possibly due to either heterogeneity within DD Type II or variable gene expression [2, 8].

8.4.2 Etiology

DD Type I and II are inherited as autosomal dominant traits with 100% penetrance [8].

8.4.3 Treatment

Patients generally have low to no caries incidence since the crowns do not show any deviation from normal with regard to color or morphology [19]. Patients show a low threshold value to pulp testing and present with pain due to the abnormal pulp condition of the teeth [19]. Due to the abnormal morphology of the roots, teeth are lost early leaving very little opportunity for treatment [2, 19, 20].

8.4.4 Note

According to Coster, "Recent mapping of genetic defects causing DGI Type II and III and DD Type II show that heritable dentin defects can be viewed as a continuum rather that an expression of different disease entities" [2]. With advances in genetic testing, we may find more interconnectedness between these heritable dentin disorders in the future.

References

1. Gartner LP (1999) Dentin. Essential of oral histology and embryology, Chapter 3, 3rd edn. Jen House, Baltimore, pp 37, 40–41
2. Coster PJ (2012) Dentin disorders: anomalies of dentin formation and structure. Endod Top 21:41–61
3. Sauk JJ, Gay R, Miller EJ, Gay S (1980) Immunohistochemical localization of type III collagen in the dentin of patients with osteogenesis imperfecta and hereditary opalescent dentin. J Oral Pathol 9:210–220
4. Gartner LP (1999) Tooth development. Essentials of oral histology and embryology, Chapter 2, 3rd edn. Jen House, Baltimore, pp 25–26
5. Takagi Y, Sasaki S (1988) A probable common disturbance in the early stage of odontoblast differentiation in dentinogenesis imperfecta Type I and Type II. Oral Pathol 17:208–212
6. Bailleul-Forestier I, Molla M, Verloes A, Berdal A (2008) The genetic basis of inherited anomalies of the teeth: part 1: clinical and molecular aspects of non-syndromic dental disorders. Eur J Med Genet 51:273–291
7. Lee SK et al (2009) A novel mutation in the DSPP gene associated with dentinogenesis imperfecta type II. J Dent Res 88(1):51–55
8. Shields ED, Bixler D, El-Kafrawy AM (1973) A proposed classification for heritable human dentine defects with a description of a new entity. Arch Oral Biol 18:543–553
9. Kim JW, Simmer JP (2007) Hereditary dentin defects. J Dent Res 86(5):392–399
10. Hodge HC et al (1940) Hereditary opalescent dentin III: histological, chemical and physical studies. J Dent Res 19(6):521–536
11. Pettiette MT, Wright JT, Trope M (1998) Dentinogenesis imperfecta: endodontic implications: case report. Oral Surg Oral Med Oral Pathol Oral Radiol Endod 86(6):733–737
12. Roberts E, Schour I (1939) Hereditary opalescent dentine (dentinogenesis imperfecta). Am J Orthod Oral Surg 25(3):267–276
13. Finn SB (1938) Hereditary opalescent dentin. I. An analysis of the literature on hereditary anomalies of tooth color. J Am Dent Assoc Dental Cosmos 25:1240–1249
14. Hodge HC, Finn SB, Lose GB, Gachet FS, Bassett SH (1939) Hereditary opalescent dentin II: general and oral clinical studies. J Am Dent Assoc 26(10):1663–1674
15. Shilpa PS, David CM, Kaul R, Sanjay CJ, Narayan BK (2012) Brittle teeth with brittle bone in a family for four generations: case report and literature review. Contemp Clin Dent 3(2):197–201
16. Abilabbos H, Al-Sineedi F (2013) Clinical manifestation and dental management of dentinogenesis imperfecta associated with osteogenesis imperfecta: case report. Saudi Dent J 25:159–165
17. Wadhawan R, Mishra S, Sharma S, Yadav P, Duhan H, Nazir S (2017) Dentinogenesis imperfecta in a four year old child: a case report. Int J Med Res 2(2):10–14
18. Malgrem B, Lindskog S, Elgadi A, Norgen S (2004) Clinical, histopathologic, and genetic investigation in two large families with dentinogenesis imperfecta type II. Hum Genet 114:491–498
19. Logan J, Becks H, Silverman S Jr, Pindborg JJ (1962) Dentinal dysplasia. Oral Surg Oral Med Oral Pathol 15(3):317–333
20. Vieira AR, Modest A, Cabral MG (1998) Dentinal dysplasia type I: report of an atypical case in the primary dentition. ASDC J Dent Child 65(2):141–144

Rare Dental Anomalies

9

9.1 Introduction

Some dental anomalies are common and will be encountered in clinical practice; however, others are rare and are unlikely to be seen. In general, the more severe or unusual the anomaly, the higher the likelihood that it is a component of a genetic syndrome or systemic disease. Identifying rare anomalies in patients should prompt further investigation to determine if they are related to a syndrome or other medical condition.

9.2 Facial (Labial) Talon Cusp

Talon cusps are accessory cusps located mostly on the lingual surface of permanent anterior teeth and rarely in primary anterior teeth (Fig. 9.1) [1]. They are

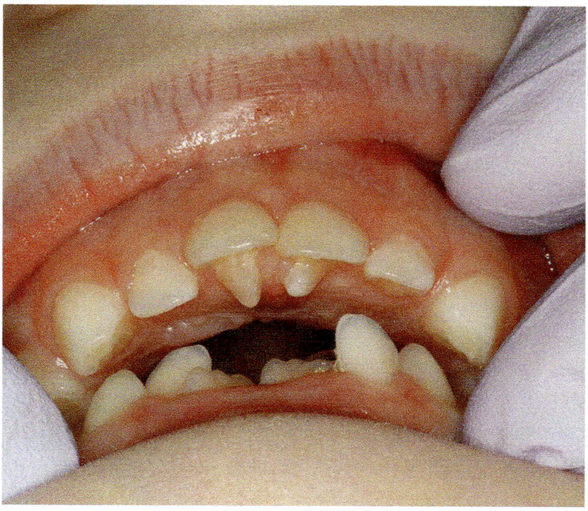

Fig. 9.1 Clinical photograph showing bilateral lingual talon cusps in maxillary primary central incisors

J. A. Soxman et al., *Anomalies of the Developing Dentition*,
https://doi.org/10.1007/978-3-030-03164-0_9

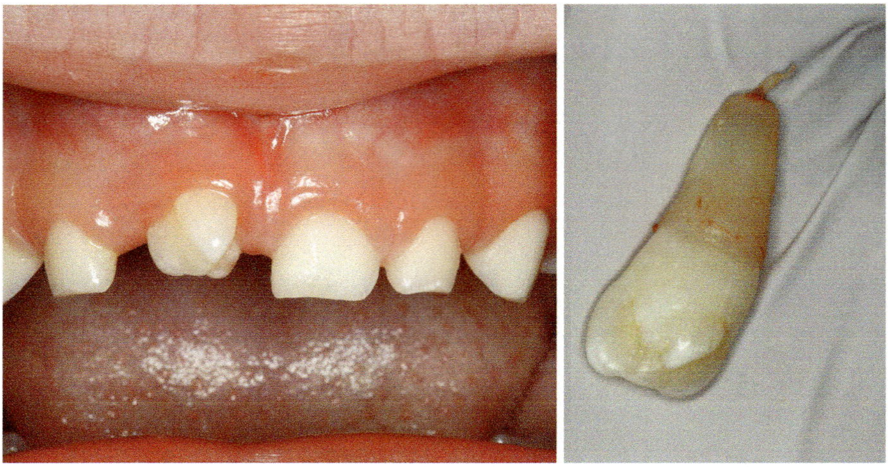

Fig. 9.2 Clinical photograph showing facial talon cusp on primary right central incisor and the extracted anomalous tooth

composed of enamel and dentin with a varying degree of pulp tissue. Talon cusps are frequently seen in syndromes like Sturge–Weber syndrome, Rubinstein–Taybi syndrome, Mohr syndrome, Ellis–van Creveld syndrome, Alagille's syndrome, Berardinelli–Seip syndrome [2, 3], and KGB syndrome [4]. It has also been reported to occur in a patient with incontinentia pigmenti achromians (IPA) [5].

The incidence of a talon cusp on the facial surfaces of anterior teeth is rare (Fig. 9.2). There are few reported cases in the literature, most in the permanent dentition but some in primary teeth [3, 6–8]. There are also reports of teeth with both lingual and facial talon cusps [9]. Clinically, facial talon cusps cause problems such as propensity of carious lesions in grooves leading to pulp pathology, soft tissue pathology, compromised esthetics, and occlusal interference.

9.3 Lobodontia

Lobodontia is a very rare, autosomal dominant dental dysmorphology in which the teeth resemble those seen in carnivores [10, 11]. The term is derived from the Spanish word *lobo* which means wolf. Dental anomalies seen are generalized microdontia, hypodontia, dens in dente, and shovel-shaped incisors [12]. The distinguishing dental features though are conical premolars and canines with accentuated cusps, giving them a "fang-like" appearance (Fig. 9.3). The molars appear multituberculate (Fig. 9.4) with single conical, pyramidal roots [11].

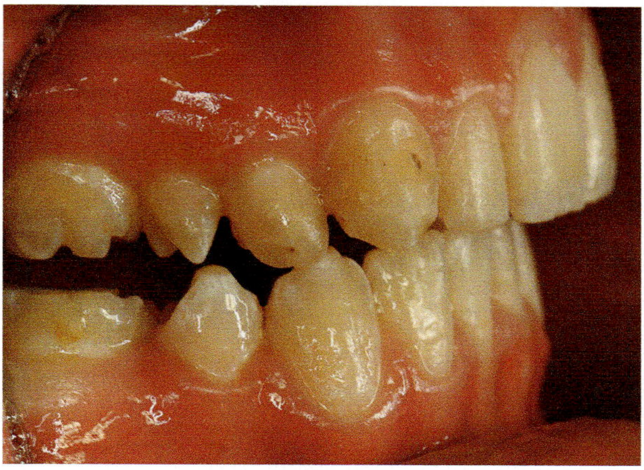

Fig. 9.3 Clinical photograph of a patient with lobodontia showing the sharply pointed canines and premolars

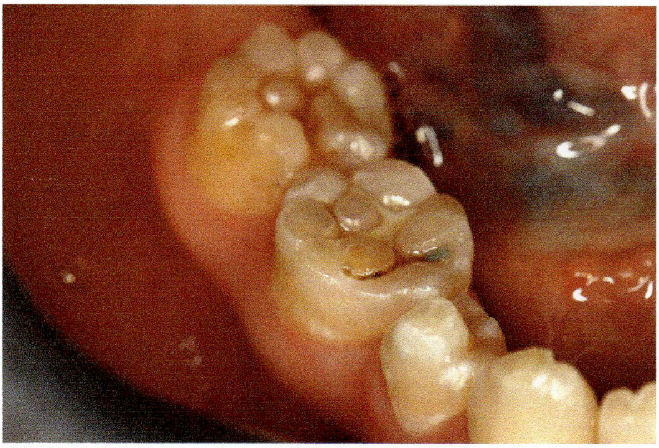

Fig. 9.4 Clinical photograph of a patient with lobodontia showing tuberculate molars

9.4 Globodontia

Globodontia refers to very large bulbous and globe-shaped crowns. It was first used by Witkop in 1976 because he noted a similarity to that of an inflated balloon [13]. They are a feature of Otodental syndrome which is an autosomal dominant syndrome with dental anomalies and sensorineural hearing loss for frequencies above 1000 Hz. It has a microdeletion at chromosome 11q13 [14, 15]. Both primary and permanent dentitions are affected. Cuspids and molars are macrodontic and have bulbous crowns (Fig. 9.5). Premolars are often missing or smaller in size, and the incisors are usually not affected. Radiographically, the affected teeth are taurodontic with a septated appearance and occasional pulp stones. The roots are usually shortened [16–18].

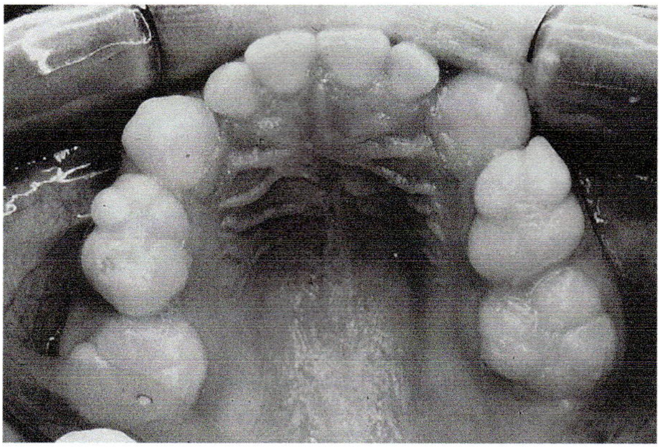

Fig. 9.5 Clinical photograph of a maxillary arch occlusal view of patient with globodontia showing the markedly enlarged canine and molar teeth (reprinted with permission from Springer Nature: Pediatr Radiol, Otodental syndrome, oculo-facio-cardio-dental (OFCD) syndrome, and lobodontia: dental disorders of interest to the pediatric radiologist, Gorlin RJ 28(10):802–4; 1998)

9.5 Radiculomegaly

Radiculomegaly, or root gigantism, is a rare dental abnormality first described by Hayward in 1980 [19]. It is a characteristic finding in oculo-facio-cardio-dental (OFCD) syndrome, which is a rare X-linked dominant syndrome [14]. This syndrome is characterized by abnormalities of eyes, face, heart, and teeth. Although other dental anomalies can be present, radiculomegaly, especially in the canines, is almost pathognomonic for this syndrome (Fig. 9.6). This condition is usually diagnosed at age 15 or later once the apices of the canines are closed. In the literature, there are only two reported cases of radiculomegaly not associated with this syndrome [20, 21].

The other dental anomalies that may be present are over-retained primary dentition, delayed permanent tooth eruption, oligodontia, hypodontia, conical-shaped teeth, macrodontia, and enamel defects (Fig. 9.7). The other features of this syndrome are cataracts, secondary glaucoma, microphthalmia, microcornea, atrial and ventricular septal defects, mitral valve prolapse, long narrow face, high nasal bridge, broad nasal tip with separation of the anterior cartilages, cleft palate, long philtrum, and laterally curved or thick eyebrows [22].

9.6 Solitary Median Maxillary Central Incisor

A solitary median maxillary central incisor (SMMCI) is a rare malformation caused by a heterozygous mutation in the Sonic hedgehog gene on chromosome 7q36. It has an incidence 1:50,000 live births and can be present as an isolated finding or associated with defects of midline structures, including the craniofacial bones, nasal

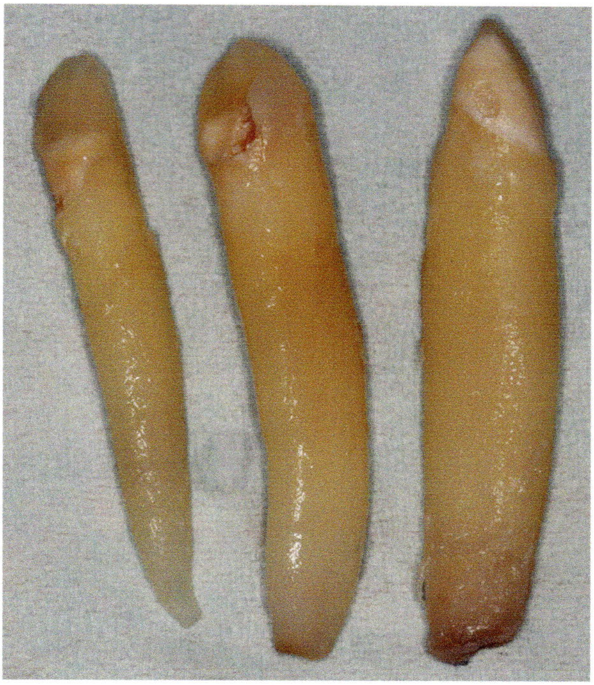

Fig. 9.6 Clinical photograph of extracted teeth showing radiculomegaly in a patient with oculo-facial-cardio-dental syndrome (OFCD)

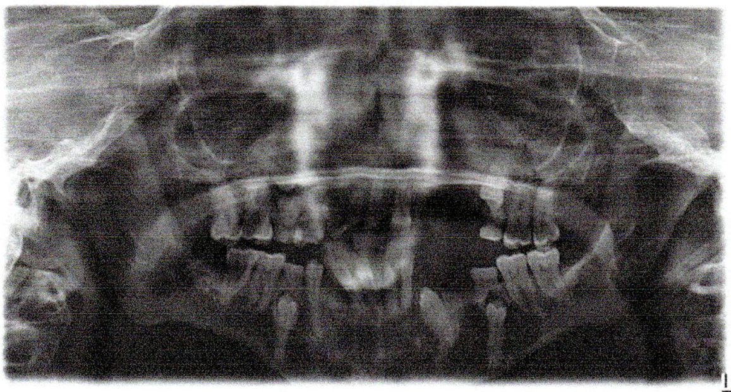

Fig. 9.7 Panoramic radiograph of patient with OFCD showing radiculomegaly of canines and premolars, delayed eruption permanent teeth, delayed exfoliation primary teeth, conical-shaped teeth, macrodontia, and hypodontia

airways, choanal atresia, nasal pyriform aperture stenosis, and the brain (holoprosencephaly) [23–25]. Other systemic alterations, such as growth hormone deficiency, short stature, mental retardation, and pituitary dysfunction, can be present. The significance of this dental midline defect is that it can be a sign or predictor of a potentially serious developmental anomaly, holoprosencephaly. This is a development defect resulting from incomplete separation of the fore brain during the embryonic period, affecting the development of anterior midline structures [26].

The most common clinical characteristic found in the oral cavity is the presence of a single central incisor at the midline of the maxilla in both primary and

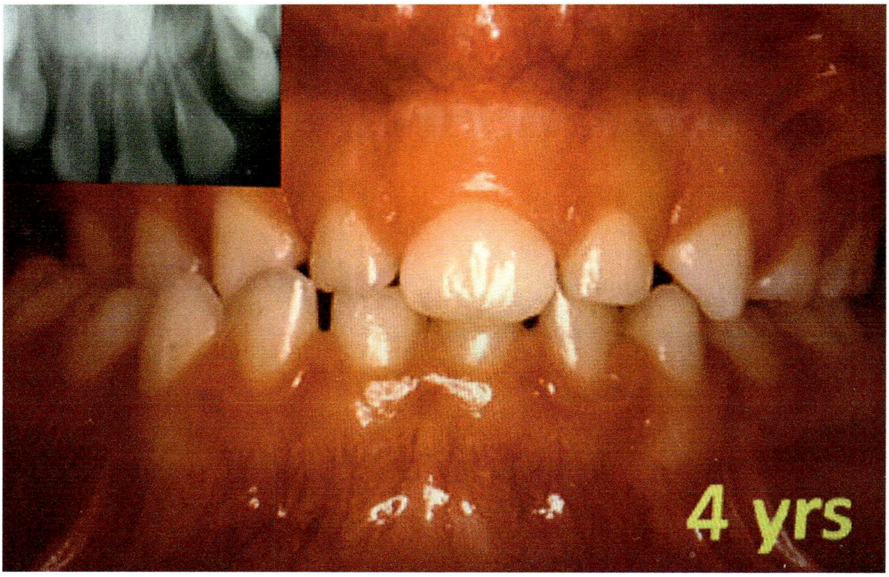

Fig. 9.8 Clinical photograph and periapical radiograph of a 4-year-old patient with solitary median maxillary incisor (SMMI) showing the presence of single midline maxillary incisor (primary and permanent) (reprinted with permission from Springer Nature: Eur Arch Paediatr Dent, Solitary median maxillary central incisor syndrome (SMMCI) with congenital nasal puriform aperture stenosis: literature review and case report with comprehensive dental treatment and 14 years follow-up Lygidakis NN, Chatzidimitriou K, Petrou N, Lygidakis NA, 14(6):417–23; 2013)

permanent dentition (Fig. 9.8) [27]. The most likely cause for this anomaly is an early defect in the frontonasal developmental field [28]. Early diagnosis of SMMCI is important, because it may be a sign of other severe congenital or developmental abnormalities and appropriate referrals for further workup are indicated.

9.7 Pyramidal Molars

Pyramidal molars (PM) have fused roots with a solitary enlarged canal (Fig. 9.9) [29]. Other terms that have been used to describe this anomaly are cylindrical, prismatic, and conical [30]. The reported prevalence for pyramidal molars is 0.5% [31], and the most commonly affected teeth are maxillary second molars. Pyramidal molars are frequently associated with taurodontism and other dental anomalies, delayed eruption, and missing or supernumerary teeth. There are also case reports describing an association between PMs with short root anomaly of the maxillary central incisors [32]. This anomaly is also seen in lobodontia as discussed above (Fig. 9.10) [33].

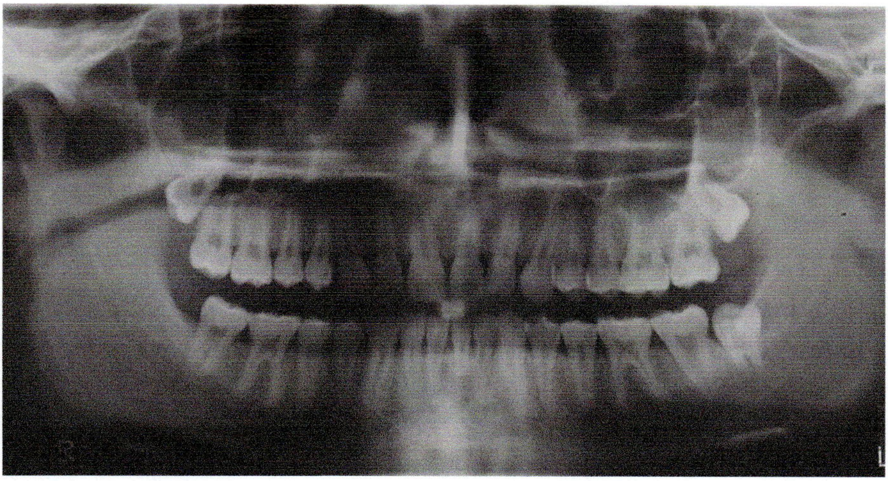

Fig. 9.9 Panoramic radiographs revealing a pyramidal molar on left mandibular second molar

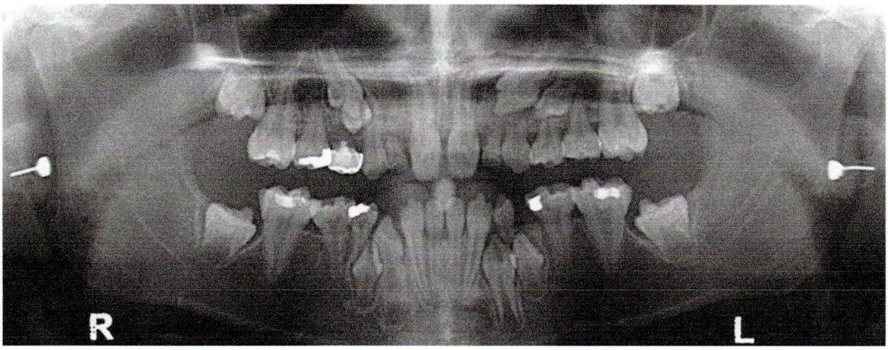

Fig. 9.10 Panoramic radiograph of patient with lobodontia showing pyramidal maxillary and mandibular molars

References

1. Hattab FN, Yassin OM, al-Nimri KS (1996) Talon cusp in permanent dentition associated with other dental anomalies: review of literature and reports of seven cases. ASDC J Dent Child 63(5):368–376
2. Ekambaram M, Yiu C, King N (2008) An unusual case of double teeth with facial and lingual talon cusps. Oral Surg Oral Med Oral Pathol Oral Radiol Endod 105(4):e63–e67
3. Sudhakar S, Madhavan A, Balasubramani S, Shreenivas S (2017) A rare familial presentation of facial talon cusp. J Clin Diagn Res 11(1):ZD15–ZD17
4. Almandey AH, Anthonappa RP, King NM, Fung CW (2010) KBG syndrome: clinical features and specific dental findings. Pediatr Dent 32(5):439–444

5. Tsutsumi T, Oguchi H (1991) Labial talon cusp in a child with incontinentia pigmenti achromians: case report. Pediatr Dent 13(4):236–237
6. Kulkarni VK, Choudhary P, Bansal AV, Deshmukh J, Duddu MK, Shashikiran ND (2012) Facial talon cusp: a rarity, report of a case with one year follow up and flashback on reported cases. Contemp Clin Dent 3(Suppl 1):S125–S129
7. Nuvvula S, Gaddam KR, Jayachandra B, Mallineni SK (2014) A rare report of mandibular facial talon cusp and its management. J Conserv Dent 17(5):499–502
8. Topaloglu Ak A, Eden E, Ertugrul F, Sutekin E (2008) Supernumerary primary tooth with facial and palatal talon cusps: a case report. J Dent Child (Chic) 75(3):309–312
9. Gallacher A, Ali R, Bhakta S (2016) Dens invaginatus: diagnosis and management strategies. Br Dent J 221(7):383–387
10. Robbins IM, Keene HJ (1964) Multiple morphologic dental anomalies. Report of a case. Oral Surg Oral Med Oral Pathol 17:683–690
11. Skrinjaric T, Gorseta K, Skrinjaric I (2016) Lobodontia: genetic entity with specific pattern of dental dysmorphology. Ann Anat 203:100–107
12. Ather A, Ather H, Acharya SR, Radhakrishnan RA (2013) Lobodontia: the unravelling of the wolf teeth. Romanian J Morphol Embryol 54(1):215–217
13. Witkop CJ Jr, Gundlach KK, Streed WJ, Sauk JJ Jr (1976) Globodontia in the otodental syndrome. Oral Surg Oral Med Oral Pathol 41(4):472–483
14. Gorlin RJ (1998) Otodental syndrome, oculo-facio-cardio-dental (OFCD) syndrome, and lobodontia: dental disorders of interest to the pediatric radiologist. Pediatr Radiol 28(10):802–804
15. Sedano HO, Moreira LC, de Souza RA, Moleri AB (2001) Otodental syndrome: a case report and genetic considerations. Oral Surg Oral Med Oral Pathol Oral Radiol Endod 92(3):312–317
16. Cehreli SB, Brannon RB, Musselman RJ, Tirali RE, Derbent M (2014) Otodental syndrome: a case presentation in a 6-year old child. Eur J Paediatr Dent 15(2 Suppl):215–217
17. Colter JD, Sedano HO (2005) Otodental syndrome: a case report. Pediatr Dent 27(6):482–485
18. Santos-Pinto L, Oviedo MP, Santos-Pinto A, Iost HI, Seale NS, Reddy AK (1998) Otodental syndrome: three familial case reports. Pediatr Dent 20(3):208–211
19. Hayward JR (1980) Cuspid gigantism. Oral Surg Oral Med Oral Pathol 49(6):500–501
20. Kemoli AM, Junior TM (2017) Bilateral second premolars agenesia together with a unilateral canine radiculomegaly. Contemp Clin Dent 8(1):151–154
21. Smith MH, Cohen DM, Bhattacharyya I, Islam NM, Kashtwari D (2018) Radiculomegaly: a case report of this rare dental finding with review of the associated oculo-facio-cardio-dental syndrome. Oral Surg Oral Med Oral Pathol Oral Radiol. https://doi.org/10.1016/j.oooo.2018.02.011
22. McGovern E, Al-Mudaffer M, McMahon C, Brosnahan D, Fleming P, Reardon W (2006) Oculo-facio-cardio-dental syndrome in a mother and daughter. Int J Oral Maxillofac Surg 35(11):1060–1062
23. Hall RK (2006) Solitary median maxillary central incisor (SMMCI) syndrome. Orphanet J Rare Dis 1:12
24. Lygidakis NN, Chatzidimitriou K, Petrou N, Lygidakis NA (2013) Solitary median maxillary central incisor syndrome (SMMCI) with congenital nasal puriform aperture stenosis: literature review and case report with comprehensive dental treatment and 14 years follow-up. Eur Arch Paediatr Dent 14(6):417–423
25. Viana Eda S, Kramer PF, Closs LQ, Scalco G (2010) Solitary median maxillary central incisor syndrome and holoprosencephaly: a case report. Pediatr Dent 32(5):424–427
26. Ilhan O, Pekcevik Y, Akbay S, Ozdemir SA, Memur S, Kanar B, Kirbiyik O, Ozer EA (2018) Solitary median maxillary central incisor, holoprosencephaly and congenital nasal pyriform aperture stenosis in a premature infant: case report. Arch Argent Pediatr 116(1):e130–e134
27. Cho SY, Drummond BK (2006) Solitary median maxillary central incisor and normal stature: a report of three cases. Int J Paediatr Dent 16(2):128–134
28. Sekerci AE, Ucar FI, Gumus H, Aydinbelge M, Sisman Y (2012) Solitary median maxillary central incisor: a report of 2 cases. Pediatr Dent 34(2):150–155

29. Ackerman JL, Ackerman AL, Ackerman AB (1973) Taurodont, pyramidal and fused molar roots associated with other anomalies in a kindred. Am J Phys Anthropol 38(3):681–694
30. Holan G, Chosack A (1991) Single-rooted molars in the primary and permanent dentition in two siblings: case report. Pediatr Dent 13(6):367–369
31. Burklein S, Breuer D, Schafer E (2011) Prevalence of taurodont and pyramidal molars in a German population. J Endod 37(2):158–162
32. Klein U, Paimagham B, Blumhagen R, Kroehl M, Sain J (2017) Pyramidal and taurodont molars and their association with other tooth anomalies. Pediatr Dent 39(1):46–52
33. Nguyen AM, Tiffee JC, Arnold RM (1996) Pyramidal molar roots and canine-like dental morphologic features in multiple family members: a case report. Oral Surg Oral Med Oral Pathol Oral Radiol Endod 82(4):411–416

Printed by Printforce, the Netherlands